100

SIMPLE THINGS

YOU CAN DO TO PREVENT

ALZHEIMER'S

And Age-Related Memory Loss

100

SIMPLE THINGS

YOU CAN DO TO PREVENT

ALZHEIMER'S

And Age-Related Memory Loss

JEAN CARPER

Vermilion
LONDON

3 5 7 9 10 8 6 4

Published in 2011 by Vermilion, an imprint of Ebury Publishing
Ebury Publishing is a Random House Group company

First published in the USA by Little Brown & Company, a division of
Hachette Book Group, Inc.

Copyright © 2010 by Jean Carper

The Random House Group Limited Reg. No. 954009

Addresses for companies within the Random House Group can be found at
www.randomhouse.co.uk

A CIP catalogue record for this book is available from the British Library

The Random House Group Limited supports the Forest Stewardship
Council ® (FSC ®), the leading international forest certification organisation.
All our titles that are printed on Greenpeace approved FSC® certified
paper carry the FSC® logo. Our paper procurement policy can be found at
www.randomhouse.co.uk/environment

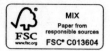

Printed and bound in Great Britain by
CPI Antony Rowe, Chippenham, Wiltshire

ISBN 978-0-09-193951-9

Copies are available at special rates for bulk orders. Contact the sales
development team on 020 7840 8487 for more information.

To buy books by your favourite authors and register for offers,
visit www.randomhouse.co.uk

To my mother, Natella Carper, 1904–2000,
an inspiring spirit who lived ninety-five years without dementia
and a final year with probable vascular dementia

And to my sisters, Joan Hickson
and Judy Stevens, with whom I share
a single copy of the ApoE4 Alzheimer's susceptibility gene

PUBLISHER'S NOTE

As stated by the author, "On many levels, Alzheimer's research is an exciting grab bag of uncertain theories, despite a hardcore center of scientific belief. Certainty about cause and preventive interventions has not yet been engraved in stone." So while this book includes preventive measures based on research by credentialed investigators, the information and advice contained in this book should not be interpreted as a definitive way to prevent Alzheimer's but rather as a guide to suggested measures that may help prevent Alzheimer's. This book is not intended to replace the services of a physician, nor does it constitute a doctor-patient relationship. Information in this book is provided for informational purposes only. You should consult your physician or health care professional regarding your care, in particular, with respect to any symptoms that may require diagnosis or medical attention. This book was current as of June 2010, and as new data become available through research, experience, or changes to product contents, some of the information in this book may become outdated. Any action on your part in response to the information provided in this book is at your discretion. You should consult your physician or health care professional concerning any information contained in this book, and follow their professional advice. The publisher makes no representations or warranties pertaining to any information contained in this book and is not liable for any direct or indirect claim, loss, or damage resulting from the use of information contained in this book.

Please note that the author is not active as an investor, owner, consultant, writer, or management participant in any nutritional supplement company or enterprise, and does not profit financially from the promotion or sale of any nutritional supplements.

CONTENTS

Contents

Contents

Contents

Contents

Contents

100

SIMPLE THINGS

YOU CAN DO TO PREVENT

ALZHEIMER'S

And Age-Related Memory Loss

WHAT TO DO WHILE WE WAIT
FOR A CURE

There's an amusing saying: "Of all the things I've lost, I miss my mind the most." For some reason, this has always slightly disturbed me, and lately more than ever. Quite accidentally, as the result of a routine blood test for cholesterol factors a few years ago, I discovered that I carry a gene that makes me exceptionally vulnerable to Alzheimer's disease. So do my two younger sisters. The gene, ApoE4, is carried by about 25 percent of Americans, and although it is not the only gene associated with Alzheimer's, it is the most dominant one so far discovered.

That doesn't mean, of course, that I or others so genetically marked are doomed to develop Alzheimer's. But knowing I have inherited this tiny time bomb, which may already be slowly and methodically deconstructing my brain cells and vaporizing my intellect, has dramatically focused my attention on ways to neutralize this threat to my aging brain.

Perhaps I have long sensed I could be a target. For nearly forty years, as a medical and nutrition writer concentrating on the predicament of aging, I have closely followed the research findings on Alzheimer's and age-related memory loss—from the increasingly exciting investigations into basic biochemical causes to the new surge of research into how to deter, slow, or even reverse the pathology and symptoms of memory loss.

As a senior medical correspondent for CNN, I did a documentary in the 1980s on the scientific quest for an Alzheimer's cure. My most memorable moment was when world-renowned Alzheimer's researcher Peter Davies, PhD, at Yeshiva University's Albert Einstein College of Medicine reached into a freezer and produced a slice of an Alzheimer's brain, given up at autopsy. It showed large holes—enlarged ventricles carved out by the disease. "Like a piece of Swiss cheese" he volunteered as he put the cold remains into my hand. The image of that diseased brain remains indelibly in my mind. I have often wondered exactly how the biological architect of disease worked to create the void that robbed that particular brain of its function and humanity, and if science would ever be able to stop or prevent the devastation that perhaps might be going on inside my own brain.

Fortunately, many researchers at leading medical centers have wondered the same thing, and applied their inventive minds to solving the Alzheimer's puzzle. Over the past twenty-five years, they have learned much about the pathology of Alzheimer's—and have spun many theories about what makes neurons get sick, become dysfunctional, and die; why brains become abnormally shrunken; and why learning and memory disappear. The pursuit of understanding the disease, of course, is a prelude to an antidote or a cure—possibly a vaccine or pharmaceutical potions that may one day magically halt the damage and perhaps even restore a dreadfully emaciated brain back to robust health.

Many experts I talk to think they will ultimately conquer Alzheimer's, which now afflicts 35 million people around the world and threatens to become a global tsunami of 115 million by 2050, as increasing life expectancy leaves us with an ever-expanding aged population.

Yet the dilemma of what to do in the meantime has not escaped Alzheimer's investigators. Many are shifting their focus to the imperative of prevention—the idea that we should try to head off the awful consequences of the disease before it transforms our brains beyond the point of no return. "It is far easier to rescue a sick neuron than a dead neuron," says prominent brain researcher David Bennett, MD, at Rush University Medical Center in Chicago. He and other leaders in the field are vigorously pursuing new ways to identify, prevent, and postpone brain changes and symptoms of age-induced neurodegeneration before they are irreversible.

Eric B. Larson, MD, and Thomas J. Montine, MD, leading Alzheimer's investigators at Seattle's Group Health Research Institute and the University of Washington, expressed that view in a recent editorial in the *Journal of the American Medical Association*. The dramatically increasing global life expectancy, they wrote, makes it "difficult to *overstate the urgency* of finding solutions that prevent, delay, slow, and treat Alzheimer's disease and related dementias."

You may be surprised to know that many researchers now see Alzheimer's and other forms of dementia as diseases of "lifestyle" as well as genetics. That may soften some of our fear and feelings of helplessness surrounding the disease. Surveys show that Americans over age fifty-five, including me, fear Alzheimer's more than any other disease, even cancer, stroke, and heart disease. At the same time, most of us subscribe to the prevailing view that we are virtually powerless to protect ourselves against a disease seemingly so mysterious and cruel as to preclude any possibility of avoiding its onset. That is understandable, but authorities now say it is mostly a myth.

Researchers are increasingly struck by the fact that Alzheimer's has some of the same lifestyle origins as heart disease and diabetes, such as obesity, high bad LDL cholesterol, high blood pressure, and physical inactivity—although admittedly, the stakes seem higher when the target is your brain. Nothing can surpass the threat of losing your entire self—your intellect, personality, or reasons for staying alive. And that acknowledgment is what makes many Alzheimer's researchers so zealous in their quest for new strategies of prevention and early intervention.

WHAT IS ALZHEIMER'S, ANYWAY?

Alzheimer's disease is the most common form of dementia (which means "deprived of mind"), accounting for 60 to 80 percent of all cases of dementia. According to strict scientific definition, Alzheimer's dementia is a slow, progressive deterioration and shrinkage of the brain, characterized by two peculiar types of neuronal damage — clumps and plaques of a sticky gunk called beta-amyloid, and tangles, formed by another brain toxin known as tau. It is decidedly a disease of aging; age is the number one risk factor. Symptoms are rare before age sixty-five. After that, your chances of Alzheimer's double every five years. About half of all people over age eighty-five have Alzheimer's, according to the Alzheimer's Association. This does not mean, however, that Alzheimer's is a part of "normal aging." Alzheimer's is a chronic disease, and abnormal memory impairment is a warning sign.

Researchers used to define Alzheimer's as a single form of dementia, but in reality it's more complicated, says Larson. It is most often an overlapping combination of Alzheimer's dementia; vascular dementia, a disease of blood vessels in the brain; and something called Lewy body dementia, characterized by protein deposits also found in Parkinson's disease. The global symptoms of all dementias are much the same: severe deficits in cognition, particularly memory, and often motor activity that interfere with normal behavior and functioning.

Your vulnerability to Alzheimer's and other dementias is influenced by your genes. But genes are not the final deciders. They can be muted or magnified and partially subdued by your lifestyle and environment. It's also important to distinguish between early-onset Alzheimer's, before age sixty, and late-onset, after age sixty. Early-onset is caused by genetic mutations and is thus quite strongly inherited, but is rare, accounting for only 5 percent of all cases. The overwhelming threat for nearly all of us is late-onset Alzheimer's, which can be influenced by so-called susceptibility genes, such as ApoE4. This means that people with these genes are more predisposed, but by no means predestined, to develop Alzheimer's. Also, it may be possible to curtail the expression of such genes early in the disease process, essentially "curing" Alzheimer's before it becomes irreversible.

Most important, researchers no longer view Alzheimer's as a sudden brain catastrophe of old age; they now see it as a continuum of disease that spans decades and is influenced by early, midlife, and late-life factors such as nutrition, infections, education, diabetes, and mental and physical activity. The impact of these lifetime influences on your brain is typically silent until you reach your sixties, seventies, and eighties. Like other chronic diseases, Alzheimer's is a long time arriving.

Twenty to thirty years of slow and surreptitious neuro-degeneration may pass before Alzheimer's brain pathology releases its symptoms to public view. Brain functioning worsens as neurons shrink and die primarily in the brain's cognitively sensitive regions, including the frontal cortex and hippocampus, prime victims of Alzheimer's.

In stunning new discoveries, made possible by brain-imaging technology and cerebrospinal-fluid analyses, scientists can now see the earliest origins of detrimental changes in the brain that produce symptoms years later. Using sophisticated PET scans, prominent researcher John C. Morris, MD, director of the Alzheimer's Disease Research Center at Washington University in St. Louis, sees deposits of toxic beta-amyloid, a hallmark of Alzheimer's, in the brains of a large percentage of older people who have yet to show any signs of mental impairment.

Morris's pioneering work documents that long before symptoms appear, there is a prolonged prelude of disguised normalcy (with seeds of destruction that show up on brain scans), frequently followed by a decade or so of gradual decline called mild cognitive impairment (MCI) or, more accurately, "early Alzheimer's disease." It is during this long time span of pre-symptomatic changes and mild impairment that he and others hope to identify the most vulnerable individuals and to use interventions to postpone the onset of Alzheimer's for many years or to prevent it entirely—which essentially means delaying serious symptoms until you die of something else.

As Maine geriatrician Laurel Coleman, MD, who sits on the board of the Alzheimer's Association, puts it, "Let's say you're dialed in to get Alzheimer's disease at eighty-two. You may be able to push that back until maybe you're ninety-two." Prominent Alzheimer's researcher Suzanne Tyas, PhD, at the University of Waterloo in Ontario, suggests it may be possible to push the symptoms of Alzheimer's so far into the future that they "don't happen until an age when most of us will no longer be alive."

The prospect of intervening to turn the clock back on

Alzheimer's has tremendously exciting implications. "It's estimated that if we could delay the onset of Alzheimer's for even five years, *it would reduce the number of new cases by half,*" says leading researcher Suzanne Craft, PhD, at the University of Washington.

YOU CAN RESCUE YOUR OWN BRAIN

As heartbreaking and devastating as Alzheimer's is, optimism is growing that we can lessen the risk and possibly save ourselves. A new slogan, entirely in sync with the latest scientific thinking, is showing up on blogs: "We have found a cure for Alzheimer's, and it is prevention." Top Alzheimer's investigators are now telling us that whether we develop the disease is not entirely random and capricious, not a matter of fate or destiny, nor an inevitable consequence of aging.

Yes, we may face an epidemic as baby boomers age, and yes, there may also be a partial or complete cure in our future. But the fact is, our susceptibility to Alzheimer's, like heart disease, cancer, and diabetes, though somewhat at the mercy of genes, is also partly influenced by factors within our control. And the disease's long lead time gives us years of opportunity in which to make a difference. Especially remarkable is that the state of your health in middle age—your forties and fifties—appears to foreshadow the health of your brain in your seventies and eighties.

Further, science clearly suggests that the daily decisions you make, even the small ones, can help build a brain able to function successfully into your nineties, or for an entire lifetime. Top scientists have documented the surprising power we have over our brains' destiny. For example, by eating the right foods, having a large social network, doing the right exercise, taking the right supplements, and controlling your blood sugar, depression, and stress, you can lower your chances of Alzheimer's, perhaps delaying it for so long that it does not become manifest during your lifetime.

Remarkable studies at the University of Washington School of Medicine find that eating a high-saturated-fat, high-sugar diet boosts brain levels of beta-amyloid, a toxic protein blamed for spreading the devastation of Alzheimer's. Eating certain other foods appears to lessen the toxic amyloid threat to brain cells. After surprising experiments, distinguished brain researcher Carl Cotman, PhD, at the University of California, Irvine, judged physical exercise more effective than any known drug in protecting the brain from damage leading to Alzheimer's and memory loss.

Especially intriguing is evidence that even severe pathology is not destiny. Some elderly brains function well even though riddled with the brain-damaging plaques and tangles consistent with a diagnosis of Alzheimer's. The explanation, suggest scientists: a particular lifestyle, which may include a higher education, a large social network, and intellectual activities, can bolster the brain's so-called cognitive reserve enough to overwhelm its physical wounds, so it appears to function normally long past the time it should. It makes you realize that nobody can predict what miracles the human brain can perform when pushed, prodded, soothed, and stimulated.

Rush University neuropsychologist Robert S. Wilson, PhD, says it best: "We now understand that brain activity depends not just on genes, but on how you live your life.... A lot of the disease we call Alzheimer's is outside plaques and tangles."

Clearly, the health of your brain, like that of your heart, is a far more personal choice than you probably realize. We all can do some things to help our brains negotiate the hazards of advancing age.

WHY THIS BOOK?

In recent years, I have noticed the increasing mountain of research on what we might do to deter and defer Alzheimer's. This research has always piqued my interest because of the genetic throw of the dice that triples my own risk. I often thought that when I had collected 100 scientifically supported possibilities for outliving and avoiding Alzheimer's and age-related memory decline, I would put them in a book to help answer this question: what do we do while we await the anticipated Alzheimer's cure?

I finally did find 100 simple things people can do to build brains that are more resistant to aging and primed to function successfully over a long lifetime. I am well aware that you may not want to try them all at once and that there are some you may never try. Think of this book as a large buffet table. You may want to sample everything in it, or again, you may not. I suggest you try anything that strikes you as interesting and appealing. It's true that some things may work better for some people than others, depending on unknown genetic differences and individual preferences. It is impossible to say at this stage of the research which things will be most effective for you, although any type of mental stimulation, regular physical exercise, social engagement, and a high-antioxidant diet seem to have the edge.

As everyone knows, science is full of surprises. For years, mainstream medicine thought that gastrointestinal ulcers were caused by diet and stress. It took an Australian physician a decade to prove to the establishment skeptics that ulcers are caused by the bacterium *Helicobacter pylori* and treatable with antibiotics. Thus I don't refrain from including some scientific theories that are on the sidelines of mainstream research. On many levels, Alzheimer's research is an exciting grab bag of uncertain theories, despite a hard-core center of scientific belief. Certainty about cause and preventive interventions has not yet been engraved in stone.

However, this book includes only preventive measures based on research by credentialed investigators, most of whom are affiliated with leading scientific institutions. Offbeat preventive ideas do not get exposure here unless they come from scientifically valid sources.

Do I religiously do all of the things I suggest in this book? Mostly, and certainly in the area of nutrition and diet. I have recently taken up tennis again after a decade of being away from it. Yoga is new for me, as is water aerobics. At this writing, I have yet to filter my drinking water, and I can't do a crossword puzzle or play Scrabble (and never could). I am hoping that writing this book has given me a major infusion of mental activity, although I have lost some sleep over it (not good for the brain). I have no trouble being social (a good thing for the brain), although by definition a writer's life means spending many hours sedentary and alone. I don't take many nature walks and probably spend way too much time at the movies, and even though I like to think that films are mentally stimulating, I have no evidence to prove it. Most important to me, my seventy-eight-year-old brain seems to be functioning reasonably well, despite my genetic handicap. And I want to keep it that way. Still, I am aware that life, like science, holds surprises. Whether Alzheimer's is waiting in my future is unknown. But I am doing my best to outlive it, and I am inviting you to do the same.

> *For a list of the main scientific references used in this book and updates on preventing Alzheimer's, go to www.jeancarper.com.*

1

GET SMART ABOUT **ALCOHOL**

It can boost
brain cells or destroy them

Your brain may like a little alcohol, but not a lot. Study after study shows that moderate drinkers are less apt to develop Alzheimer's. Recent research at Wake Forest University Baptist Medical Center found that older people who drank eight to fourteen alcoholic beverages per week—one or two a day—had a 37 percent lower risk of dementia than nondrinkers. The bad news: stepping into the "heavy drinker" category—more than fourteen drinks a week—doubled the odds of developing dementia compared to not drinking.

UCLA researchers find that heavy drinking pushes you two to three years closer to Alzheimer's. And heavy drinkers who also carry the ApoE4 Alzheimer's gene can expect the onset of dementia four to six years earlier. Further, in the large Framingham Heart Study, a community health study spanning several decades, heavy drinking (more than fourteen drinks a week) predicted shrinkage in the memory regions of the brain.

British doctors writing in the *British Journal of Psychiatry* recently warned that heavy and binge drinking among older people is creating "a silent epidemic" of alcohol-related dementia that causes as much as 10 percent of all cases of dementia.

Even adults who usually drink lightly or moderately but go on occasional binges face a higher risk of dementia. A Finnish study showed that adults who binged in midlife at least once a month—drinking, for example, more than five bottles of beer or a bottle of wine at one sitting—were three times more likely to develop dementia, including Alzheimer's, twenty-five years later. Passing out from alcohol at least twice in one year hiked the chances of developing dementia by ten times.

On the other hand, a daily cocktail or glass of wine may help delay dementia. Research finds that alcohol is an anti-inflammatory (inflammation promotes Alzheimer's) and raises good HDL cholesterol, which helps ward off dementia. High antioxidants in red wine give it additional anti-dementia clout. Such antioxidants, including resveratrol, act as anti-coagulants and artery relaxants, dilating blood vessels and increasing blood flow, which encourages cognitive functioning. That makes many researchers favor red wine over white wine, which has comparatively few antioxidants. (See "Make It Wine, Preferably Red," page 282.)

What to do? Understand that alcohol in low doses over an adult's lifetime appears brain protective, but large doses at one time kill or cripple brain cells, leaving you more vulnerable to cognitive dysfunction and Alzheimer's decades later. The toxic impact is long lasting. If you do drink, stick to low or moderate amounts, sipped slowly, preferably with food. That means no more than one drink a day for women, two for men. One drink usually means a twelve-ounce beer, a shot of liquor, or five ounces of wine.

2

CONSIDER **ALPHA LIPOIC ACID AND ALCAR**

These two supplements work together to rejuvenate your aging brain

If you could take one antioxidant to ensure good cognitive functioning as you age, what would it be? The answer seems clear to prominent researchers at Oregon State University's Linus Pauling Institute. Alpha lipoic acid, also known as lipoic acid, is the strongest antioxidant rejuvenator of aging brains we have ever seen in aged animals, says institute researcher Tory Hagen, PhD, noting that it's especially powerful when combined with the supplement acetyl-l-carnitine (ALCAR).

Hagen has pioneered the study of lipoic acid and ALCAR, along with biochemistry professor Bruce Ames, PhD, at the University of California, Berkeley. Now eighty, Ames discovered ALCAR in the 1990s being sold as a "smart drug" in Italy. In groundbreaking research, he and Hagen showed that old, sluggish rats became as physically and mentally active as rats half their age within a few weeks of being fed ALCAR and lipoic acid. "It's like a seventy-five-year-old having the energy of a forty-year-old," says Ames.

He explains that brain cells require ALCAR as fuel to keep tiny energy generators called mitochondria humming along. As we age, we synthesize 50 percent less ALCAR. Deficient in fuel, our cellular energy factories become dysfunctional and leave neurons sputtering in disorganized communication. Mitochondrial distress in brain cell synapses is one of the earliest biochemical clues that Alzheimer's is on the march, according to recent research. Boosting ALCAR in brain cells helps revive mitochondrial functioning, creating a surge in overall mental and physical energy, claims Ames. ALCAR also blocks the formation of Alzheimer's tau tangles in test tubes.

The critical job of alpha lipoic acid in brain cells is to stand guard over the mitochondrial energy plants, protecting them against damage from the continual onslaught of free-radical chemicals. Lipoic acid is one of the few known antioxidant molecules able to zip through the blood-brain barrier to fend off such destruction. Lacking the antioxidant protection found in lipoic acid, the mitochondria factories tend to collapse and shut down, leaving your brain in a constant state of "brownout."

Hagen also discovered another way lipoic acid appears to prevent and reverse brain damage. It "chelates," or flushes, iron deposits out of the brain. As you age, iron accumulates in neurons and accelerates the "oxidative damage" blamed for cognitive decline and dementia. After Hagen fed old rats high doses of lipoic acid for just two weeks, the iron in their brains dropped dramatically to the levels normally seen in young rats.

In humans, alpha lipoic acid has been shown to help lower blood pressure, blood sugar, and triglycerides; reverse insulin resistance; and prevent diabetic neuropathy. Some doctors routinely give 600 milligrams of lipoic acid a day to diabetics to help prevent complications.

What to do? Consider taking either or both of these supplements to boost brain-cell functioning. You can find them separately and together in health food stores or drugstores and online. If you buy ALCAR alone, be sure the label says acetyl-l-carnitine and not just plain L-carnitine.

Both alpha lipoic acid and acetyl-l-carnitine are considered safe at the recommended daily doses of 200 mg per day for lipoic acid and 500 mg per day for ALCAR, although you can take lower doses if you want. If you take higher doses to address a medical problem, such as diabetes, do so only with the advice and monitoring of a health professional.

The University of California, Berkeley, has patented a combination pill of 200 mg of alpha lipoic acid and 500 mg of aceytl-l-carnitine, the doses recommended by Ames. It is called Juvenon and is available at http://juvenon.com. Ames says he donates any money he receives from its sale to human testing of the supplement. Several other companies market combinations of lipoic acid and ALCAR.

3

ASK QUESTIONS ABOUT **ANESTHESIA**

Could anesthesia bring on Alzheimer's?

I t's not uncommon to be in a mental fog when you come out of surgery. Typically, the anesthesia wears off quickly, although it can linger for days or weeks. On occasion, doctors see cases like the sixty-five-year-old woman who, six months after hip surgery, develops memory loss and is later diagnosed with Alzheimer's. Is it coincidence? Or could anesthesia cause permanent damage, accelerating the onset of Alzheimer's — especially in those genetically susceptible or already suffering the mild cognitive loss that precedes dementia?

The possibility worries some experts. Roderic G. Eckenhoff, MD, a professor of anesthesiology at the University of Pennsylvania School of Medicine in Philadelphia, says, "We give these drugs to millions of patients every year and blithely ignore that they could have long-term effects." He notes that lab animals subjected to common inhaled anesthetics show increased death of brain cells, detrimental clumping of toxic beta-amyloid and tau, and long-lasting cognitive dysfunction, including memory loss. Eckenhoff fears that such anesthetics may accelerate the onset of dementia and Alzheimer's, especially in vulnerable elderly brains.

So does Rudolph Tanzi, PhD, a renowned Alzheimer's genetics researcher at the Massachusetts General Hospital in Boston. He, as well as Eckenhoff, has focused on the hazards of isoflurane, a widely used general anesthetic. Their experiments show that isoflurane makes beta-amyloid activity in cell cultures more toxic and lethal. Their theory: if an elderly brain has deposits of amyloid, as most do, exposing it to isoflurane makes it worse, possibly hastening Alzheimer's. Research also suggests that individuals carrying the ApoE4 gene may be particularly susceptible to harm from isoflurane.

Tanzi advocates avoiding isoflurane if possible. When his mother recently had surgery, he asked the anesthesiologist to substitute desflurane, another inhaled anesthetic, for isoflurane. As quoted in *Forbes* magazine, Tanzi explained, "We don't have enough data yet to ban isoflurane, but I'm convinced enough that I won't let my mother have it. I would advise any family or friends to stay away from isoflurane. There is a lot of speculation here, and a lot of work needs to be done, but at this point I wouldn't take a chance."

In contrast, a recent Washington University study did *not* find permanent cognitive problems among a large group of surgery patients, suggesting that anesthesia may not be a brain danger, but some experts say the jury is still out. According to a University of Washington study, just being hospitalized for a critical or noncritical illness also boosted an older person's odds of dementia.

What to do? Right now, without expert agreement, it is unclear how much patients getting anesthesia need to worry. Reported postsurgical cognitive problems and irreversible memory loss seem to affect mainly older people who are particularly susceptible to Alzheimer's. Some researchers advise patients to talk over any concerns with their anesthesiologists. In any event, you should be aware of the potential problem and alert for the results of further research.

4

CHECK OUT YOUR **ANKLE**

Low blood flow in your foot is a clue to trouble in your brain

A surprisingly simple, noninvasive, inexpensive test can reveal the cognitive state of your brain and your likelihood of stroke and dementia. It involves an ultrasound device called a Doppler along with a blood-pressure cuff that compares systolic blood pressure in your ankle with that in your arm. It's called an ankle-brachial index (ABI) test and takes about fifteen minutes to perform in your doctor's office.

The theory: blood vessel health is similar throughout the body. The degree of clogged arteries and blood flow in the feet predicts the degree of atherosclerosis in cerebral blood vessels. This quick test, then, is a measure of generalized atherosclerosis. Its primary use is to detect peripheral artery disease, or PAD, in the lower limbs, but studies have shown that it is also amazingly accurate in picking up on cognitive impairment in older people and the possibility of stroke and Alzheimer's.

Researchers at the University of Edinburgh tracked more

than seven hundred older men and women ages fifty-five to seventy-four, for ten years. Those with the lowest ABI readings, signifying blood flow impairment, scored 60 to 230 percent lower on tests of reasoning, verbal fluency, and information-processing speed. Conclusion: the ABI test identified older individuals at higher risk of cognitive impairment.

In a National Institute on Aging study of over twenty-five hundred elderly men, those with low ABI readings were 57 percent more likely to develop Alzheimer's and 225 percent more apt to suffer from vascular dementia within the next eight years. Vascular disease, as detected by the ABI test, shows up in the cerebral arteries as blockages, loss of brain tissue, and inflammation—all likely causes of cognitive decline and dementia.

Further, the test spots people likely to have a stroke, says Souvik Sen, MD, director of the University of North Carolina Stroke Center, so they can take precautions to intervene before stroke symptoms occur.

What to do? Ask your doctor about having an ankle-brachial index test to alert you to memory problems ahead. Then, depending on the results, follow your doctor's advice on what you need to do to remedy any impairment of blood flow. That may include stepped-up exercise, strategies to control blood pressure and cholesterol, a change in diet, or medication. It's better to be forewarned of future cognitive trouble when you can do something to prevent it than to find out later, when you cannot.

5

DON'T SHY AWAY FROM **ANTIBIOTICS**

Amazingly, they may help guard against Alzheimer's

Why do some people with Alzheimer's become more lucid after taking antibiotics? The stories are so legendary that doctors cannot disregard them.

Here are two anecdotes from the daughters of Alzheimer's patients posted on the online nonprofit Alzheimer Research Forum, an interactive website for Alzheimer's researchers and others interested in the disease.

Case one: An elderly woman with Alzheimer's was near death and taken to an emergency room, where she was given an antibiotic drip for lung congestion. She had a mental revival that astounded her daughter: "She recognized us, was able to put three words together, and understood and responded to everything we said to her. She has not been this responsive in close to a year! I attribute it to the antibiotic drip."

Case two: A man with Alzheimer's had a serious bladder infection. According to his daughter, "The urologist gave him powerful antibiotics. After a few days on these antibiotics, my father became lucid for over a week. He did not know my name before; now he was calling me by name again and actually carrying on a conversation with me. He died about ten days later. I just thought that someone should know."

Understandably, seeing a loved one's brain come alive again is an inexplicable and shocking event. But Brian J. Balin, PhD, a professor at the Center for Chronic Disorders of Aging, Philadelphia College of Osteopathic Medicine, says that he often hears such stories of cognitive recovery after patients have taken antibiotics, and he's not really surprised.

Balin is a leading authority behind the unorthodox theory that infections are a cause of Alzheimer's. The fact that many people with the disease regain mental faculties after taking antibiotics is partial support for the theory. Indeed, a recent study showed that giving Alzheimer's patients two antibiotics, doxycycline and rifampin, for three months slowed their rate of cognitive decline.

However, antibiotics are not a permanent solution. As soon as they are stopped, the mental improvement disappears, says Balin. He thinks it highly unlikely that antibiotics can permanently reverse longtime Alzheimer's pathology. However, he speculates that antibiotics taken in mid- to late life before symptoms appear might help arrest or delay the onset of Alzheimer's.

What to do? Right now, of course, nobody is suggesting taking antibiotics specifically to ward off Alzheimer's, since no one knows if they do work, if they are safe, and which ones might be effective. The main message is to be aware that antibiotics may be brain protective and not to shy away from taking them when they are warranted to fight a specific infection. They may do more good than is currently understood. On the other hand, avoid excessive exposure to antibiotics that are not clearly needed to combat a particular illness.

6

EAT **ANTIOXIDANT-RICH FOODS**

They are powerful antidotes to memory decline

There's almost universal scientific agreement: eating certain foods infuses your brain with compounds called antioxidants that can slow cognitive decline and help prevent Alzheimer's. It's been documented in aging people, old dogs, and countless lab animals.

Here's why: Every time you breathe, you take in oxygen, which sparks formation of free-radical chemicals. These chemicals can run amok, ripping cell membranes, mutating DNA, blocking synapses, and disrupting neural communication networks. Such devastation is called "oxidative damage" or "molecular rust." Your brain is a prime target of free radicals because it is fatty and burns so much oxygen. When oxidized, the fat in your brain literally becomes rancid, like spoiled meat. Such ongoing damage accelerates cognitive dysfunction and possibly Alzheimer's.

That's where molecular soldiers called antioxidants come in. They zip around the brain, capturing and snuffing out rampaging free radicals. These determined terminators, always on patrol, create a formidable and versatile defense system against brain degeneration. And where do you recruit antioxidants? From specific foods, mostly fruits and vegetables. Tests at Tufts University noted that blood antioxidant capacity surged after test subjects ate ten ounces of fresh spinach or eight ounces of strawberries.

Never underestimate the power of two or three carrots, broccoli florets, or spinach leaves. Among a group of older people, eating three servings of vegetables a day slowed the rate of memory decline by 40 percent, compared to eating less than one serving of vegetables a day, according to researchers at Chicago's Rush Institute for Healthy Aging. A Harvard study of aging women found particular cognitive-function-preserving antioxidant power in green leafy vegetables (spinach, kale, and lettuce) and cruciferous vegetables (broccoli, cabbage, cauliflower, and Brussels sprouts). Columbia University researchers found that the best anti-Alzheimer's foods are antioxidant heavy hitters, including tomatoes, cruciferous vegetables, dark and green leafy vegetables, fruits, salad dressings, nuts, and fish. New Yorkers over age sixty-five who ate the most of those foods, and the least high-fat dairy products, red meat, organ meat, and butter, were 38 percent less likely to develop Alzheimer's.

What to do? Never miss a chance to eat a fruit or vegetable to infuse your brain with antioxidants. Five to nine daily portions are great, but know that every little bit counts. It's crazy to starve your brain cells of ammunition that could prevent a takeover by Alzheimer's.

Foods vary in their concentration of total antioxidants and types. Deep color is a tip-off. That's why berries are tops. Be sure to include the edible skins of fruits and vegetables. For example, 31 percent of the antioxidants in a red delicious apple is in its skin, and you lose 40 percent of a cucumber's antioxidants if you peel it.

Here, in order, are 30 fruits and vegetables (juices excluded) with the greatest antioxidant capacity, based on weight, according to a 2010 analysis of 326 selected foods by the U.S. Department of Agriculture. If one of your favorites is not on the list, eat it anyway. It's bound to have some antioxidants. Not all fruits and vegetables have yet been properly tested.

1. Black raspberries
2. Elderberries
3. Raisins, golden
4. Blueberries, wild
5. Artichokes
6. Cranberries
7. Dried plums (prunes)
8. Black currants
9. Plums
10. Blackberries
11. Garlic
12. Red raspberries
13. Blueberries, cultivated
14. Strawberries
15. Dates
16. Cherries
17. Figs, raw
18. Red cabbage
19. Apples with peel
20. Leaf lettuce, red
21. Pears with peel
22. Asparagus
23. Sweet potatoes
24. Broccoli rabe and florets
25. Oranges
26. Beet greens
27. Avocados
28. Red grapes
29. Radishes
30. Spinach

7

KNOW ABOUT THE ApoE4 GENE

It dramatically increases your chances of getting Alzheimer's

One in four of you reading this has a specific genetic time bomb that makes you three to ten times more susceptible to developing late-onset Alzheimer's, which typically occurs after age sixty. The gene is called apolipoprotein E4, or ApoE4. If you inherit a single variant of ApoE4 from one parent, your Alzheimer's risk triples. If you inherit a double dose of ApoE4 from both parents, your risk rises by ten times or more.

Here's the simple reality: Carrying ApoE4 does not doom you to Alzheimer's, but it is the number one known genetic threat. Lots of people with the ApoE4 gene never get Alzheimer's. Lots of people without ApoE4 do get it. About 40 percent of all Alzheimer's patients are ApoE4 positive, according to the National Institute on Aging. And ApoE4 carriers are likely to get the disease earlier and to have more severe brain atrophy than noncarriers.

Recent surprising evidence from brain scans and cognitive tests reveals that people with the ApoE4 gene show signs of brain damage (deposits of beta-amyloid) and memory decline much earlier than previously believed—between the ages of fifty-five and sixty, according to leading researcher Richard Caselli, MD, and colleagues at the Mayo Clinic in Arizona, who compared carriers with noncarriers.

Finding such early age-related memory decline in ApoE4 carriers is extremely significant, says Caselli. He believes it signals "the initiation point of Alzheimer's at which people go from being normal to starting to be abnormal." It also has important implications in the effort to prevent Alzheimer's. It argues for starting interventions in midlife, at ages forty to fifty, the time when research shows such risk factors as cholesterol, obesity, diabetes, and blood pressure are most predictive of Alzheimer's. Also, much research shows that preventive strategies differ in effectiveness depending on whether you have the ApoE4 gene.

The obvious question: Should you know your ApoE4 status? Cardiologists sometimes test for it because it influences blood cholesterol. Doctors may be reluctant to order the test to identify Alzheimer's susceptibility, fearing the knowledge could be psychologically crippling. However, a study at Boston Medical Center found "no harm" among a group of healthy adults given the news of their ApoE4 risk, according to senior author Robert C. Green. In fact, recognizing their increased vulnerability to dementia and heart disease caused some to ratchet up their exercise regimens.

What to do? Unless knowing your ApoE4 status would cause you anxiety, it may make sense to find out so that you can use the knowledge to lower your Alzheimer's risk. It entails a simple blood test of ApoE isoforms, and you can ask for it when you have your blood cholesterol checked. Or ask your doctor about a DNA test specifically to reveal your ApoE genotype.

If you are ApoE4 positive, doing most of the things in this book may help deter Alzheimer's, but studies suggest you are likely to particularly benefit from taking folic acid daily; avoiding head injuries; restricting saturated fats; eating lots of anti-oxidants; exercising regularly; and building extensive "cognitive reserve" through higher education, mental stimulation, and physical and social activity. Unfortunately, ApoE4 carriers may not get as much anti-Alzheimer's benefit from eating fatty fish, taking high-omega-3 fish oil capsules, or drinking red wine as noncarriers.

8

DRINK **APPLE JUICE**

It may mimic an Alzheimer's drug

Call it "natural Aricept." Apple juice can boost the production of acetylcholine in the brain, which is the same thing the number-one-prescribed, highly advertised pharmaceutical drug Aricept (donepezil) does to treat Alzheimer's, according to recent research. Scientists have known for forty years that brains racked by Alzheimer's are typically short on the neurotransmitter acetylcholine, essential for forming memories and learning. Thus it makes sense to stimulate nerve cells to produce more, pumping up memory and slowing mental decline. That's what Aricept is designed to do. And, surprisingly, it's also what apple juice does, say researchers at the University of Massachusetts, Lowell.

Scientists spiked the drinking water of old mice with apple juice concentrate. Sure enough, the production of acetylcholine in their brains picked up. More surprising, says lead researcher and cellular neurobiologist Thomas Shea, PhD, was their increased speed and accuracy on memory and learning tasks, such as maneuvering their way through mazes. He credits the surge in acetylcholine in nerve cells induced by the apple juice. How much juice did the mice get? The human equivalent of two 8-ounce glasses of juice or two to three apples a day for a month, says Shea.

He explains that apple juice hypes acetylcholine by supplying antioxidants, mainly quercetin, that prevent damage to neurons from free-radical chemicals. Also exciting, test tube studies show that apple juice may help curb the brain buildup of beta-amyloid deposits responsible for bringing on Alzheimer's.

What to do? Go with the old adage that an apple a day (make that two apples or two cups of juice) keeps the doctor—in this case, the geriatric neurologist—away. A brain bonus: apples also help fight inflammation; reduce the risk of type 2 diabetes, high blood pressure, stroke, and gum disease; and promote a smaller waist—all factors in Alzheimer's disease. No kidding. According to a government analysis, people who down a cup of apple juice, a large apple, or a cup of applesauce a day are 21 percent more apt to have a slimmer waist, and that means less chance of developing Alzheimer's.

9

BEWARE OF **BAD FATS**

It's scary to see how they destroy brain cells

Scientists have known for at least twenty-five years that animals allowed to gorge on bad fats become "dumb and dumber." Pioneering researcher Carol Greenwood, PhD, at the University of Toronto has long documented the horrific damage that bad fats, notably saturated animal fats and trans fats, can inflict on your brain and intellect. As she says, "It's scary."

After consuming the same percentage of saturated animal fats as in a typical American diet, her lab animals developed severe brain and memory dysfunction. The more they ate, the less they could remember. On a diet of 10 percent saturated fat, the animals learned virtually nothing.

Bad fats affect human brains the same way, accelerating the onset of memory decline and Alzheimer's. Martha Clare Morris, ScD, at Rush University in Chicago found that elderly people who ate the most trans fats were four times more likely to develop Alzheimer's than those eating the least. Eating the most saturated fats more than doubled their likelihood of Alzheimer's. In a large government study, older women who ate the most trans fats (7 grams a day) were 30 percent more likely to suffer a stroke than women who ate the least (1 gram a day).

Incredibly, the type of fat you eat changes your brain's architecture and functioning for better or worse. Saturated fats strangle cerebral cells; membranes stiffen and shrivel; dendritic tentacles that communicate with other cells become stunted; neurotransmitters dry up or become short-circuited. Toxic beta-amyloid, a hallmark of Alzheimer's, piles up.

Consequently, damaged brain cells become inefficient and dysfunctional, leading to diminished memory and learning abilities.

Another alarming way saturated fats cause memory decline is by predisposing a person to insulin resistance, a dysfunctional condition implicated in type 2 diabetes and Alzheimer's. Insulin resistance is considered the main link that makes diabetics so vulnerable to Alzheimer's. It can definitely lead to memory impairment, says Greenwood. Millions of Americans suffer from insulin-related memory problems, most without suspecting that eating bad fats is a big part of the reason.

On the other hand, omega-3 fish oil and monounsaturated fats (such as olive oil) make brain cells smarter and more efficient and less prone to Alzheimer's.

What to do? Think of saturated fats and trans fats as brain enemies and stay away from them as much as possible. Restrict fatty meats, which also destroy cognitive function in other ways. Buy low-fat or fat-free dairy products, including milk, cheese, and ice cream. Trim skin from poultry. And run like crazy from trans fats. Check for trans fats on the labels of processed foods, including chips, doughnuts, cookies, crackers, stick margarine, solid baking fats, and salad oils. Cut down on deep-fried foods; leave them in the supermarket and at fast-food restaurants. (Also see "Yes, Yes, Yes—Eat Fatty Fish," page 124, and "Go for Olive Oil," page 222, and "Beware of Omega-6 Fat," page 224.)

10

KEEP YOUR **BALANCE**

Good balance slashes your odds of developing dementia

How long can you stand on one leg? That simple test of balance helps reveal how likely you are to develop Alzheimer's. A study at the University of Washington found that a decline in physical balance was one of the first signs of future dementia, even before impaired memory.

Researchers tested the physical functioning of 2,288 people age sixty-five or over with no signs of dementia. After six years, 319 had developed dementia. Main message: those with the best balance and walking abilities at the start of the study were *three times less likely* to have developed dementia as those with lower physical functioning.

Similarly, among people who have mild memory impairment, as many do after age sixty, those with good balance also showed a slower rate of progression to full-blown Alzheimer's, according to a recent Italian study. Poor balance predicts a faster decline if you develop dementia. In a French study, Alzheimer's patients who could not stand on one leg for more than five seconds had over twice the rate of decline in tests of memory and cognition.

Starting at around age forty, your balance begins to decline for two main reasons: a loss of strength in the ankles, legs, and hips, and a progressive failure of the vestibular system, which controls equilibrium, due to subtle brain damage.

Normally, people ages thirty to seventy should be able to stand on one leg for 30 seconds with their eyes open and their arms crossed on their chest; between ages seventy and seventy-nine, for 28 seconds; and after eighty, for 21 seconds, says Marilyn Moffat, PhD, a professor of physical therapy at New York University. A truer test of balance as you age is to stand on one leg with your eyes closed, adds John E. Morley, MD, a professor of geriatrics at St. Louis University School of Medicine. It's usually surprising how much worse your balance is without visual cues. At first, most people over seventy can't stand on one leg with eyes closed for more than several seconds. But the good news is, practicing can dramatically improve your balance within a couple of weeks or months, according to Morley and Moffatt. The more you do exercises to improve balance, the better it gets, they say.

How long should you be able to stand on one leg with eyes closed? Charts vary, but "normal" is reported to be 24 to 28 seconds before age fifty, 21 seconds from ages fifty to fifty-nine; 10 to 20 seconds from sixty to sixty-nine; 4 to 9 seconds from seventy to seventy-nine, and 4 seconds or less after that.

What to do? Be sure to include exercises to maintain and improve balance in your daily routine, especially after age sixty. Advice from the Mayo Clinic: "Try balancing on one foot while waiting in line, or stand up and sit down without using your hands." Also work on specific balance exercises at your gym, or check with local senior centers and hospitals to see if they conduct classes in balance. Moffat says that adults of all ages should make it a goal to stand on one foot, eyes open, for at least 30 seconds. Morley puts it this way: "Regardless of your age, if you can't stand steadily on one leg for at least 15 seconds—with or without eyes closed—then you definitely need to start practicing as soon as possible to improve your balance." If you practice at home, be sure to stand near a countertop or table where you can catch yourself, or have someone nearby to catch you. Don't risk falling.

Also consider tai chi; a month or two of tai chi can improve balance, research shows. Yoga is also known to benefit balance. Two excellent books with examples of exercises to improve balance are *Age-Defying Fitness* by Marilyn Moffat and Carole B. Lewis and *The Science of Staying Young* by John E. Morley and Sheri R. Colberg. You can also find exercises on the National Institute on Aging's website, www.nia.nih.gov/exercise.

11

EAT **BERRIES** EVERY DAY

They may help prevent and reverse mental and physical aging

Imagine, compounds in berries actually get into your brain cells and accumulate there. They improve how neurons behave, how well they communicate, and whether they become inflamed and dysfunctional or rejuvenated, vital, and alert. Truly, scientists regularly witness how much better aging brains function when fed berries of all types.

James Joseph, PhD, and Barbara Shukitt-Hale, PhD, neuroscientists at Tufts University, were astounded to see old, cognitively damaged animals suddenly regain memory, balance, and motor skills after eating blueberries, blackberries, raspberries, strawberries, and cranberries. "They just get younger and smarter," they observed. In other experiments, the researchers prevented cognitive decline in aging animals by feeding them berries. "Eating berries will never cure Alzheimer's," they concluded, "but we are convinced they may prevent it or at least delay its onset."

Even small amounts of berries may help keep aging memory intact. Alzheimer's researchers at Rush University Medical Center in Chicago found that older women who ate strawberries at least twice a month had a 16 percent slower rate of cognitive decline.

The main secret to berries' power to protect neurons and stimulate cognitive functioning is their high content of polyphenols and anthocyanins, antioxidants revealed by berries' deep, intense colors. Such compounds block brain-cell-destroying oxidative damage and inflammation, underlying causes of Alzheimer's, and even help stimulate the birth of new brain cells. Berry chemicals may also help overcome genetic susceptibility to Alzheimer's, researchers say.

A couple of anti-Alzheimer's bonuses: berries contain chemicals that discourage weight gain and also fight infections, such as *Helicobacter pylori*, which may be associated with Alzheimer's.

What to do? Do as the brain researchers who study berries do: eat at least a half cup and preferably a cup or more every day — fresh, frozen, or as juices and in smoothies. That includes blueberries, strawberries, raspberries, blackberries, black currants, boysenberries, and cranberries. And mix them: the dominant compounds in each have different benefits for brain cells. If you eat dried berries, check the label for added sugar.

Blueberry researcher Robert Krikorian, PhD, at the University of Cincinnati, advises buying frozen berries year-round; freezing occurs within several hours of harvesting and fully preserves the nutritional and antioxidant benefits. He suggests microwaving the berries for ten to twenty seconds just before eating instead of leaving them out to thaw, which can diminish their antioxidant potency.

12

GROW A **BIGGER BRAIN**

More brain mass helps you survive
Alzheimer's damage

The bad news is: normally your brain starts to shrink when you reach thirty or forty, so it takes longer to learn, retain, and recall new information during the trip to old age. If massive numbers of neurons die off in specific brain regions involved in cognitive functioning, Alzheimer's could be in your future. But the exciting good news is: you can grow new brain cells and pump up the size and functioning of old ones precisely in those brain regions that govern memory and learning. In short, you can grow a bigger, more efficient brain that may help fend off Alzheimer's.

Scientists used to say it was impossible for the brain to regenerate. Then landmark discoveries by Fred Gage, PhD, at the Salk Institute for Biological Studies in California, and by other researchers showed that thousands of neurons are born in the brain daily, primarily in the hippocampus, a learning and memory region. The process is called neurogenesis. Neuroscientists now know that by encouraging the birth and survival of these nascent neurons, you can increase the size and intellectual strength of your brain, making it more resistant to memory decline and dementia.

Undeniably, increased brain mass equals superior cognition. The hippocampus of old people with sharper memories was 20 percent larger than that of those with poor cognition, despite similar Alzheimer's pathology, according to research at Oregon Health and Science University. Johns Hopkins University researchers found "enlarged hippocampal neurons" in the brains of deceased elderly nuns who had remained intellectually sharp, although autopsies showed severe Alzheimer's-type damage. Researchers believe the plumper neurons with more synapses (communication centers) sprang from thinking, reading, and an active mental and social life. This subtle neuronal growth helps explain the power of so-called cognitive reserve, the brain's ability to suppress symptoms of Alzheimer's, despite extensive pathology. (See "Build 'Cognitive Reserve,'" page 77.)

And what stirs your neurons to reproduce and sprout new connections? Activity. Gage was blown away when he noticed that brain cells rapidly *doubled* in mice given access to a running wheel. Studies show a brisk walk every day stimulates the birth and growth of brain cells. Brain scans reveal that only six months of aerobic exercise (walking), but not nonaerobic exercise (stretching, toning, and strengthening), increased gray matter in elderly brains.

The very act of learning—but only if it takes effort—

keeps newborn neurons alive. Taxi drivers who memorize extensive maps of a city have more gray matter than normal drivers. Living in a stimulating environment and practicing meditation are associated with larger brain volume.

People who consume lots of vitamin B_6 and B_{12} have greater brain volume. Omega-3 fish oil stimulates neuronal birth. So does increased brain blood flow. Chocolate and berries may help grow a bigger brain. Having high self-esteem and a feeling of control over your life also indicate a larger hippocampus, say researchers at McGill University in Montreal.

On the other hand, many things lead to abnormal brain shrinkage, hastening the onset of memory loss and Alzheimer's. Among them are obesity, chronic stress, B-vitamin deficiencies, longtime heavy drinking, inflammation, and sleep deprivation, along with physical and mental inactivity.

What to do? Avoid a lifestyle and activities that shrink your brain—those that may lead to excessive alcohol, stress, overweight, nutritional deficiencies, and loss of sleep. Involve your brain and body in extensive physical, social, and mental activities. That means think, study, learn new things, walk, dance, work out, and have meaningful relationships with family and a broad circle of friends. And be sure to get regular aerobic exercise, which some experts say is the surest antidote to brain atrophy associated with Alzheimer's. Pay attention to your diet and weight. Don't miss a chance to build a bigger, more resilient brain to cope with Alzheimer's pathology in case it shows up.

13

CONTROL **BLOOD PRESSURE**

It's a prime way to slow down or prevent dementia

Keeping your blood pressure normal in midlife and old age is increasingly recognized as a major deterrent to dementia. "Hypertension is at the top of the list of things that we can prevent that lead to cognitive decline in the elderly," says Dr. Walter Koroshetz of the National Institute of Neurological Disorders and Stroke. In fact, uncontrolled high blood pressure instigates early memory loss, doubles your odds of Alzheimer's, and boosts vascular dementia risk six times.

No doubt about it, high blood pressure is an underlying menace behind multiple brain catastrophes that trigger both Alzheimer's and vascular dementia.

One of the most dreaded is "brain attack," or stroke. High blood pressure more than doubles a man's chances of stroke, says Harvard research. And the higher the pressure, the greater the likelihood of stroke. For each 10 mm Hg increase in systolic pressure (the top number), odds of an ischemic (blood clot) stroke go up 28 percent, and 38 percent for a hemorrhagic, or bleeding, stroke.

If you had an MRI of your brain, you might see evidence of tiny microbleeds or clots, called mini-strokes, as well as patches of white, indicating "scarring," both resulting from high blood pressure and leading to memory loss and cognitive dysfunction.

Then there is insidious damage that spreads through the brain, called vascular dementia, in which tiny blood vessels in the brain are diseased or clogged, shutting off oxygen and glucose to brain cells. When enough cells wither or die, so does memory. High blood pressure initiates much of the damage to blood vessels that leads to vascular dementia.

A stronger predictor of dementia is high systolic blood pressure—over 140 mm—in midlife, according to National Institute on Aging research. However, high blood pressure is still a dementia risk into your eighties and nineties. In fact, a study at the University of Western Ontario estimated that controlling high blood pressure in individuals over age eighty with specific cognitive problems would prevent half of them from progressing to dementia.

The good news: taking blood pressure drugs can dramatically lower the likelihood of dementia. However, research disagrees on which types are most effective. Experts at the University of Texas School of Public Health in Houston who recently reviewed the evidence singled out ACE inhibitors and diuretics as the best proven hypertensive drugs for reducing dementia risk and progression. A large Boston University study of eight hundred thousand patients, mostly male, over age sixty-five found that taking both ACE inhibitors and angiotensin receptor blockers (ARBs) to control blood pressure slashed the risk of Alzheimer's by half. Another large study at Wake Forest University School of Medicine in North Carolina concluded that only the type of ACE inhibitors that are "centrally acting" (penetrate the brain) prevent cognitive decline.

What to do? Do everything to keep blood pressure down—preferably under 120 systolic over 80 diastolic—starting early in life. Blood pressure equal to or greater than 140 systolic and 90 diastolic is considered too high. Check your blood pressure regularly with a home monitoring device. If it is consistently high, consult a doctor for advice.

Effective strategies: Cut salt intake. Go on the DASH diet (page 88). Exercise. Give up sugary soft drinks; more than two and a half a day raised high-blood-pressure risk 87 percent in one study. Take up meditation. (A recent study in the *American Journal of Hypertension* shows that practicing Transcendental Meditation reduces high blood pressure significantly.) Take appropriate blood-pressure-lowering drugs as prescribed by your doctor; their impact can be huge in keeping your brain dementia-free.

14

GET A QUICK **BLOOD-SUGAR TEST**

Find out now if you are on a fast track for Alzheimer's

High circulating blood glucose is a sign that memory loss and Alzheimer's may be in your future. Millions of people are borderline or over the top and don't suspect it. Good news: You no longer have to get a full-blown fasting or oral glucose-tolerance test to find out. You can now discover your risk in less than ten minutes after a mere finger prick. It is called the A1c test, now the recommended standard way to screen for diabetes, according to a radical change in procedure by the American Diabetes Association.

Most important, the A1c test reveals not just your blood sugar level at the time of the test, but the average level over the previous two to three months, giving a much more accurate picture of risk. Typically, a lab technician pricks the tip of your finger, squeezes out a few drops of blood, puts it in a machine for six or seven minutes, and reads the number (or sends the sample off to a lab for analysis). Between 4 and 6 percent is normal; 6.5 percent or over indicates diabetes, and between 6 and 6.5 percent signals prediabetes, at high risk of developing diabetes.

Here's how it works: Too much glucose in your blood sticks to, or "glycates" with, hemoglobin, a protein that carries oxygen to cells. The A1c test measures the percentage of glycated hemoglobin in the bloodstream, reflecting how well your body generally is controlling glucose.

High circulating excess glucose is quite harmful and presages damage to many organs and systems, including the brain. Recent discoveries show a direct link between high blood sugar and the development of Alzheimer's. Some experts even call Alzheimer's "diabetes of the brain."

What to do? Don't wait until memory problems occur and diabetes sets in. Find out now the status of your blood sugar, so that if it is high, you can take immediate action to lower it before it harms your brain. The American Diabetes Association advises *everyone* age forty-five and over to get this blood sugar test. And it's especially critical if you are overweight or have a large waist size, high blood pressure, abnormal lipid levels, or a family history of diabetes. Asking your doctor for this quick A1c blood sugar test is one of the easiest, most important things you can do to save yourself from cognitive decline and Alzheimer's.

15

BE A **BUSY BODY**

Literally, the more you move, the better you think

You would expect planned physical activity—walking, running, swimming, engaging in sports, working out at the gym—to boost your brain. But what about that all-day-long mundane stuff? Getting out of bed, brushing your teeth, opening the refrigerator door, making coffee, taking a shower, dressing, shaving, putting on makeup, driving a car, using a computer, making a sandwich, running a vacuum, fidgeting while waiting in line…well, you get the idea—all the little movements of daily activity.

The surprising good news: these tiny movements can add up to big cognitive dividends. Researchers at the Alzheimer's Disease Center, Rush University in Chicago, had more than five hundred normal subjects in their eighties wear a wristwatch-size device called Actical for ten days. This amazing little gadget records the degree and intensity of every physical activity, from traditional vigorous exercise to small muscle movements.

It stores the information as "activity counts." Adding up the "activity counts" over twenty-four hours gives you an extremely accurate measure of your "total daily activity."

Researchers then compared the subjects' "total daily activity" levels with their cognitive test scores. Remarkably, higher "total daily activity" predicted higher cognitive functioning on all five of these important measures: episodic memory, semantic memory, working memory, perceptual speed, and visuospatial abilities. And this was true regardless of age, sex, education, weight, vascular diseases, or other factors tied to dementia.

This exciting information gives new meaning to using physical activity to fight off Alzheimer's, say researchers. Traditional exercise is still critically important, but in the interim, you can rack up benefits by virtually any imaginative way you can think of to move your muscles.

What to do? Anything that keeps your body busy. Keep your foot jiggling, your fingers fidgeting; use stairs wherever you can. Just remember to move those muscles—little ones, big ones, whenever and wherever. As far as your brain knows, all activity counts to help deter memory loss and possibly Alzheimer's.

For more information about Actical to track total daily activity, go to www.minimitter.com. You can find other "physical activity monitors" on the Internet, including the Gruve (www.gruve.com), a device developed in cooperation with the Mayo Clinic.

16

DON'T BE AFRAID OF **CAFFEINE**

It might keep Alzheimer's toxins
out of your brain

Imagine. Caffeine may not just prevent Alzheimer's; it also promises to help clean up the mess the disease has already started, according to remarkable new research by Gary W. Arendash, PhD, a research professor at the Florida Alzheimer's Disease Research Center. That means if your memory is already showing signs of decline, caffeine may help resurrect it by actually removing some of the toxic stuff causing brain damage.

Arendash added caffeine to the drinking water of mice genetically prone to Alzheimer's from middle to late life, when they typically show signs of dementia. The caffeine equaled five cups of coffee a day for humans. Guess what? The mice on caffeine did *not* show classic dementia behavior or brain changes. They performed just as well on cognitive tests as normal mice of the same age.

Moreover, the caffeine-fed mice had less Alzheimer's-creating beta-amyloid deposits in their brains. That's when

Arendash concluded that caffeine did not just modify minor factors, such as inflammation. Caffeine struck directly at the disease process, by shrinking the deposition of amyloid in the brain by an astonishing 50 percent! Caffeine works by suppressing enzymes that make toxic amyloid, he explains.

He pressed his luck further by giving caffeine-spiked water to old mice already in the throes of Alzheimer's and memory loss. Within five weeks, their memory and cognitive performance improved, and brain deposits of toxic beta-amyloid shrank! This implies that caffeine washed away established plaque, rejuvenating brain structure and consequently memory and other mental functioning.

Naturally, since coffee is a major source of caffeine, Arendash drinks plenty of it, four to five cups a day—or 400–500 mg of caffeine, the amount he says is needed to protect against Alzheimer's. "It's safe, inexpensive, and at least in our Alzheimer's mice, it's as effective as anything the pharmaceutical companies have devised," says Arendash.

Although Arendash says "decaf coffee" does not reduce toxic beta-amyloid in animals, other research suggests that decaf coffee also has brain benefits, possibly because of coffee's antioxidants. (See "Say Yes to Coffee," page 74.)

What to do? If you feel comfortable with high doses of caffeine, you may want to consider getting 400 or 500 mg a day to help ward off memory loss and Alzheimer's. You can also buy 200 mg caffeine tablets and break them in two for a "one cup of coffee" 100 mg dose, says Arendash. Other common caffeine sources: tea (one third as much as coffee), cola, and energy drinks, such as Red Bull.

Be aware that individuals respond differently to caffeine and it can have drawbacks, such as anxiety, jitters, insomnia, headaches, and increased blood pressure. Drink caffeinated drinks early in the day if you tend to have insomnia. People with uncontrolled high blood pressure and pregnant women should not consume a lot of caffeine, says Arendash. Doctors may also advise certain heart patients to limit caffeine. If you are unsure whether high doses of caffeine are okay for you, consult your doctor. Or for some of coffee's brain-protecting benefits minus the caffeine, drink decaf.

17

COUNT **CALORIES**

Eat less to remember more

If only people could cut down on calories, their rate of brain aging would slow, resulting in bigger, better-functioning brains with less Alzheimer's pathology. Countless studies of mice, rats, and monkeys who sacrificed a full stomach for science have proved it's true. Feeding lab animals only 70 percent of normal calories for most or all of their lives has produced fantastic benefits.

Rhesus monkeys on a lifelong restricted-calorie diet had dramatically less age-related brain atrophy (shrinkage) in certain regions of the brain than monkeys on normal diets, found leading researcher Richard Weindruch, PhD, at the University of Wisconsin, Madison. Similarly, when researchers at Mount Sinai School of Medicine fed monkeys a low-carbohydrate calorie-restricted diet for a lifetime, their brains had fewer sticky beta-amyloid deposits, a characteristic sign of Alzheimer's.

More alarming, excessive calories actually produced memory loss and destroyed brain tissue in young rats in experiments at the National Institute on Aging. After three months, rats free to gorge at will exhibited severe memory deficits and amazingly, at postmortem, had only *half* as many brain cells as rats on a restricted-calorie diet. Columbia University researchers found that people who ate the most daily calories over a four-year period had 50 percent higher odds of developing Alzheimer's than those who ate the fewest calories.

Not surprisingly, several studies suggest that people who cut calories improve aspects of memory and have less brain inflammation and lower blood pressure and insulin dysfunction, all factors in promoting Alzheimer's.

What to do? Curb calories, because excesses lead to overweight, obesity, diabetes, and high blood pressure, all culprits in hastening brain aging and Alzheimer's. In fact, merely processing calories may cause cumulative oxidative damage in brain cells. It's a good lifestyle strategy to resist eating more calories than you need, even in early and midlife.

Important: Experts do not recommend that frail elderly people or those with Alzheimer's reduce calories in efforts to improve memory or retard the disease. It is too late to be effective and aggravates weight loss and undernourishment, which can be worse problems in the old than overeating. The point is that restricting calories earlier in life may delay deterioration of the brain in late life. This is a preventive strategy, not a treatment.

18

WATCH OUT FOR **CELIAC DISEASE**

Surprise, a wheat allergy could
poison your memory

What if you could cure memory problems by simply cutting grains from your diet? It can happen. Israeli doctors recently found that two women previously diagnosed with Alzheimer's actually had an inherited autoimmune disease, an allergy to gluten in grains known as celiac disease. The women were put on a gluten-free diet—no wheat, rye, barley, or oats. Miraculously, their memories came back. Their "Alzheimer's" disappeared.

Mistaking symptoms of celiac disease for Alzheimer's is hardly rare. Doctors at the Mayo Clinic in Rochester, Minnesota, were recently surprised to find so many elderly celiac patients with dementia and cognitive decline. Again, a gluten-free diet reversed memory loss and other cognitive problems in some, but not all, cases.

Although celiac disease, or "gluten intolerance," is linked to neurological problems, doctors often don't look for it in older patients because it's considered a childhood disease. That's changing, but not fast enough to spare countless older people the misery of living with potentially reversible dementia and other ills, says Yoav Lurie, MD, formerly at Sorasky Medical Center in Tel Aviv. Actually, most new celiac cases, he says, are now being diagnosed at ages forty or fifty. Fully a third of those diagnosed with celiac in one study were over sixty-five.

Still, in a recent survey, only 32 percent of family physicians in the United States were aware that celiac is common in adults. Canadian gastroenterologists at the University of British Columbia have suggested that older people with unexplained signs of dementia be screened for celiac disease.

What to do? It may be a shot in the dark, but ask your doctor to test for celiac (a blood test, and a biopsy of the small intestine if warranted) if you suspect a connection with memory loss, especially if accompanied by typical celiac symptoms: gas, diarrhea, stomach pain, and weight loss. The cure is a lifelong gluten-free diet. And don't forget that adults of all ages and children with mysterious gastrointestinal distress should also be tested. It could prevent a lifetime of suffering, including needless cognitive decline and dementia.

19

TREAT YOURSELF TO **CHOCOLATE**

It boosts blood circulation in your brain

When doctors at Harvard Medical School get behind chocolate, you know it's not a myth. Yes, the fact is, eating chocolate may help save your aging brain.

Cocoa, the main ingredient in chocolate, has sky-high concentrations of antioxidants called flavanols, which possess strong heart- and brain-protecting properties. For example, Scottish researchers found that eating a little over a <u>half ounce</u> <u>a day</u> of dark chocolate containing <u>500 mg</u> of cocoa flavanols (Acticoa, from the Belgian chocolate maker Barry Callebaut) for two weeks reduced blood pressure significantly. At least three studies suggest that consuming chocolate may help prevent strokes. Chocolate also has anti-inflammatory and anti-coagulant properties.

And the most dramatic discovery: drinking flavanol-rich cocoa increases blood flow to the brain. That's major because over time, a gradual slowdown of blood flow can starve the brain of oxygen and nutrients, resulting in structural damage, cognitive decline, and dementia. MRIs commonly detect low cerebral blood flow in Alzheimer's patients. Also exciting: increasing cerebral blood flow appears to stimulate the regeneration of nerve cells and the creation of new ones, a process known as neurogenesis. In short, maintaining excellent blood flow to the brain is incredibly important in slowing cognitive decline and dementia.

When Harvard Medical School professor Norman Hollenberg, MD, had people ages fifty-nine to eighty-three drink two cups of cocoa daily, each containing 451 mg of flavanols, blood flow to their brains increased an average of 8 percent after one week and 10 percent after two weeks. (Hollenberg used a high-flavanol cocoa mix called Cocoapro, supplied by Mars, Inc.)

Additionally, Johns Hopkins University researchers have found that eating dark-chocolate flavanols may lessen the severity of a stroke. Mice fed a modest dose of a chocolate flavanol called epicatechin had significantly less brain damage after a stroke than mice not fed the chocolate compound. Researchers explain that the epicatechin ensconced in the mouse brains acted as an antidote by bucking up the nerve cells' own defenses against damage. "Even a small amount of the chocolate compound may be sufficient" to jump-start the extra neuronal action that blunted the damage, researchers theorized.

What to do? Choose dark chocolate high in flavanols and low in calories and fat. Cocoa powder has the most flavanols, says chocolate authority Joe Vinson, PhD, a professor of chemistry at the University of Scranton in Pennsylvania. It has twice as many flavanols as dark chocolate, which has twice as many as milk chocolate. White chocolate has zero. You can get a rough idea of the flavanol content from the percentage of cocoa solids listed on the label; very high is 70–80 percent, says Vinson. Stay away from "Dutched" chocolate products, he advises; they are processed with alkali, which depletes antioxidants. An occasional dark-chocolate bar is okay, generally equal in flavanols to a glass of red wine. But candy also packs fat, sugar, and calories. Your best bet: make drinks using a high-flavanol cocoa mix, water or nonfat milk (hot or cold), and little or no sugar or sugar substitute.

Mars offers a very-low-calorie cocoa mix called CirkuHealth, similar to that used in Hollenberg's studies. The company says two or three cups of cocoa made with the mix provide roughly 900 mg of flavanols, the amount found to increase cerebral blood flow. It is available at www .CirkuHealth.com.

20

CONTROL BAD **CHOLESTEROL**

High levels in midlife boost odds of Alzheimer's

You're in your forties. You find out your blood cholesterol is high. You probably know it could mean heart disease ahead. You may not know it also predicts Alzheimer's, according to the largest study ever done on the subject.

Researchers at Kaiser Permanente's Division of Research and the University of Kuopio in Finland collected data for over four decades on nearly ten thousand men and women. Their conclusion: high total cholesterol (240 mg/dL or higher) in midlife increases the risk of Alzheimer's later in life by 66 percent. Even borderline-high cholesterol (200–239 mg/dL) in midlife pushes up risk of old-age vascular dementia by 52 percent.

The main point, say researchers, is that high total cholesterol (the sum of LDL, HDL, VLDL, and IDL cholesterol) is an early warning sign that appears three or four decades before dementia does. Thus, it's important to get cholesterol down in midlife rather than waiting until old age, when it may be too late to stop or reverse its harm to the brain. In fact, it's uncertain whether high cholesterol in old age (after age seventy) is still a brain threat. One study found that among men over age sixty who were not on cholesterol-lowering drugs, a ten- to fifteen-year gradual decline in total blood cholesterol actually predicted dementia.

Researchers can't really explain how high cholesterol contributes to Alzheimer's. They theorize that too much cholesterol promotes the production of toxic beta-amyloid, a hallmark of Alzheimer's; depletes antioxidants in the brain that would ordinarily block amyloid damage; and/or incites a cascade of inflammation that destroys brain tissue.

Also important: the most likely culprit in Alzheimer's, as in heart disease, is so-called bad cholesterol, LDL (low-density lipoprotein)—the one you want less of. On the other hand, the HDL (high-density lipoprotein) type, known as good cholesterol, can help save your brain, so you want more of it. (See "Raise Your Good HDL Cholesterol," page 135.)

What to do? Pay attention to harmful cholesterol early in life. Get the bad type down and the good type up. That means a heart-healthy Mediterranean-type diet—low in saturated fat and trans fats, with lots of fish, fruits, vegetables, and whole grains—aerobic exercise, normal weight, and, if required, cholesterol-lowering drugs. (See "Follow the Mediterranean Diet," page 186, and "Investigate Statins," page 242.)

21

EAT **CHOLINE-RICH FOODS**

Choline is an Alzheimer's vaccine for babies and a boon to aging brains

A woman can dramatically reduce her children's risk of Alzheimer's by eating eggs and other choline-rich foods when she is pregnant, declares prominent researcher Steven Zeisel, MD, at the University of North Carolina. In his words: "If you have a good memory in old age, thank your mother."

Astonishing as it seems, a developing fetal brain exposed to a little extra choline, an amino acid, has better structure, wiring, and intellectual capacity for an entire lifetime, says Zeisel. He and other investigators discovered that by studying lab animals. In one experiment, Duke University researchers fed pregnant rats normal amounts of choline, extra choline, or no choline. The rats fed extra choline produced offspring with superefficient, better-wired brains and "excess memory capacity," spurring them to learn faster, both in early life and as adults. Rats denied choline in utero had sluggish brains and impaired memory.

More remarkable, when the offspring with the superior choline-fortified brains grew old, their cognitive abilities did not diminish. *The rats with brains supplied extra choline in utero did not experience the normally expected age-related deficits!* Their brains were protected from the typical neurodegeneration associated with declining memory and Alzheimer's.

To function optimally, the brain needs a constant supply of choline throughout life. Aging brains fizzle without it. For one thing, nerve cells require choline to synthesize the "memory" neurotransmitter acetylcholine, which dries up in Alzheimer's brains. Choline also fends off two major villains associated with memory decline: inflammation and high levels of homocysteine. New evidence identifies choline as an important anti-Alzheimer's ingredient in the Mediterranean diet. Researchers at the University of Athens report that Greeks who ate the most choline (more than 310 mg daily) had 22 percent lower blood concentrations of C-reactive protein, a prominent sign of inflammation, than those who ate the least choline (less than 250 mg a day).

Americans are alarmingly deficient in choline. Less than 10 percent of us get enough. Your body does not produce it. The only way to get enough is through food and supplements.

What to do? Be sure to eat enough choline: at least 550 mg a day for men and 425 mg a day for women (450 mg when pregnant and 550 mg when breast-feeding). Eating eggs is an easy way to get a choline fix, says Zeisel. One large egg yolk contains about 125 mg of choline. Don't worry about eating eggs: they don't raise blood cholesterol or foster heart disease in most people. Other good sources of choline are wheat germ, peanuts, pistachios, cashews, almonds, shrimp, fish, meat, and, among vegetables, spinach, cauliflower, and Brussels sprouts.

You can also take supplements of choline, straight or as lecithin, also called phosphatidylcholine. Check the labels of lecithin supplements to be sure they provide the desired amount of choline.

22

GO CRAZY FOR **CINNAMON**

It invigorates wimpy insulin—and more

Your brain may be getting wrecked because your insulin, a hormone supposed to energize your cells with glucose, is an underachiever. Consequently, your brain can become starved of glucose and overloaded with malfunctioning insulin, creating chaos, including catastrophic rises in the toxic protein beta-amyloid, a sticky gunk blamed as a major cause of Alzheimer's.

So, what can the oh-so-common spice cinnamon do about it? Actually, quite a bit, insists Richard Anderson, PhD, an expert on diabetes at the U.S. Department of Agriculture. He found that eating cinnamon can invigorate weak, inefficient insulin, enabling it to process sugar normally. That's a big deal, because about 80 million Americans have wimpy insulin, technically called "insulin resistance," a sign of diabetes and prediabetes. Yet many don't suspect it and unwittingly expose their brain cells to progressive degeneration.

Anderson was surprised at how powerful cinnamon was

at reversing insulin resistance. In one test, he found that diabetics who ate a quarter teaspoon of cinnamon twice a day for forty days reduced their fasting blood sugar by up to 29 percent, reflecting a remarkable surge in insulin's power to process glucose. A bonus: the cinnamon also cut triglycerides by up to 30 percent and cholesterol by as much as 25 percent.

It's not magic. Anderson has identified cinnamon's most active secret ingredient—a chemical called methylhydroxy chalcone polymer (MHCP). In test tubes, MHCP increased insulin's processing of blood sugar by 2,000 percent, or twentyfold. Cinnamon also slows the digestion of high-sugar foods. In Swedish subjects who spiked their bowls of rice pudding with two and a half teaspoons of cinnamon, blood sugar levels rose only half as high after ninety minutes as levels in those who ate plain rice pudding without cinnamon.

Even more dazzling: Anderson's latest research shows that cinnamon may stop the genesis of Alzheimer's. In brain cell studies, a water-soluble cinnamon extract blocked the formation of "tau filaments," which help to initiate Alzheimer's. Anderson was more astounded to discover that the cinnamon extract, when incubated in test tubes with tau tangles, quickly destroyed them. "The cinnamon just broke them up," he says. Anderson can't say for sure that cinnamon would prevent or get rid of tau in human brains cells, but he is optimistic. He takes the cinnamon extract himself.

What to do? To help ensure against weak insulin, which may eventually bring harm to your brain cells, add cinnamon to all kinds of foods and drinks. A total of one half to one teaspoon a day is plenty for most people. You can also get a high dose of the active ingredients by taking a standardized water-soluble extract of cinnamon as a dietary supplement. Two patented brands of cinnamon extract supplements that grew out of Anderson's research are Cinnulin PF (www.cinnulin.com) and CinSulin, which includes chromium and is distributed widely in retail outlets. What dose? "At least 250 mg twice a day, but 500 mg twice a day is better," says Anderson.

23

SAY YES TO **COFFEE**

It has many ways of protecting your brain

Coffee, once considered the drink of the unhealthy, is now emerging as a tonic for the aging brain, as well as a deterrent to several chronic diseases that promote Alzheimer's. Moreover, several studies suggest that coffee drinking earlier in life reduces the risk of dementia and Alzheimer's. In one large Finnish study men and women who drank the most coffee—three to five cups per day—during middle age were 65 percent less likely to develop Alzheimer's twenty years later.

What's coffee's secret? It's anti-inflammatory, helps block the ill effects of cholesterol in the brain, and cuts the risks of stroke, depression, and diabetes, all promoters of dementia. It's also high in antioxidants and caffeine, both strong players in brain biochemistry.

But don't think coffee is all about caffeine. The amazing truth: coffee, not fruits and vegetables, is America's number one source of antioxidants. Thus, coffee is on the job continually, fighting to stop neuronal death and carrying out multiple responsibilities to lessen diabetes, high blood pressure, and strokes that bring on dementia.

Studies show that women who regularly drank two or three cups of coffee a day, *decaf or caffeinated,* cut stroke risk by 10 to 20 percent. Risk of type 2 diabetes dropped by about one-third in people who drank more than three or four cups of coffee a day, *with or without caffeine,* compared with non–coffee drinkers. Harvard experts say coffee may improve insulin sensitivity, helping account for the dramatic reduction in diabetes.

Then there's coffee's main psychoactive constituent, caffeine. To some researchers, caffeine is the major brain-protecting hero in coffee. Mind-blowing studies at the University of South Florida suggest that pure caffeine, the amount in five cups of coffee, can both prevent and partially erase dementia-causing damage in old mice by ridding their brains of beta-amyloid toxins. (See "Don't Be Afraid of Caffeine," page 56.)

What to do? If you like coffee and it likes you, go for it. Here are wise words from the Mayo Clinic: "For most people, it appears that a moderate daily intake of coffee—two to four cups—doesn't seem to hurt and may even help." Coffee with caffeine can have drawbacks if you have anxiety, heart irregularities, certain stomach problems, or insomnia. If you are caffeine intolerant, listen to your body. If you tend to have insomnia, drink caffeinated coffee early in the day. If you are pregnant, avoid or restrict caffeine.

BUILD **"COGNITIVE RESERVE"**

Fill up your brain with lots of fascinating stuff

I f you constantly pack enough interesting stuff into your brain when you are young, old, and all the years in between, you may not notice if it is taken over by the pathology of Alzheimer's. You may simply ignore the symptoms of Alzheimer's longer and act as if they don't exist or matter; never mind that PET scans show your brain as a wasteland of plaques, tangles, and other trash.

That's a concept called "cognitive reserve"; it's studied by noted neuroscientists at places like Columbia University in New York and Rush University Medical Center in Chicago. The theory explains the irrationality of how a brain crippled by Alzheimer's can be overruled by a skull full of mementos, or "reserves," collected by your brain over a lifetime. Those reserves are things like education, marriage, socializing, a stimulating job, language skills, and plenty of leisure activities—life experiences that let you masquerade as cognitively normal when your brain isn't.

The number of people who manage to live with brains wrecked by Alzheimer's without showing it is truly astonishing. Up to 25 percent of older people with full-blown pathology don't show symptoms on cognitive tests, according to British investigators. U.S. studies find that one-third of normal older people with no signs of dementia actually have brain damage warranting a diagnosis of Alzheimer's.

Amazingly, PET scans often reveal a living brain riddled with toxic beta-amyloid, yet the person whose skull it occupies exhibits little or no cognitive impairment. Experts attribute this disconnect to the power of the individual's high cognitive reserve to override the expression of pathology.

You start building cognitive reserve as a child and continue throughout life. It reflects a combination of all of your life experiences, according to Yaakov Stern, PhD, of Columbia University College of Physicians and Surgeons, an authority on cognitive reserve. All the stimulating goodies you give your brain add up and even potentiate the benefits of one another. Thus, cognitive reserve is not fixed or static; you can enlarge and empower it at any time of life.

It never seems to quit. Stern found that elderly people who engaged in the most activities, either intellectual (reading, playing games, going to classes) or social (visiting with friends and relatives), had a 38 percent lower risk of dementia than those less mentally and socially active. After reviewing twenty-two studies on the subject, Australian researchers concluded that having high cognitive reserve cuts the odds of being diagnosed with Alzheimer's by 46 percent, nearly in half!

How does it work? Researchers speculate that brains with more cognitive reserve are more efficient; one study associated better brain blood flow with greater cognitive reserve. Also, perhaps people with more cognitive reserve have developed additional neural pathways to compensate for their brain damage. For example, older people activate more areas of the brain when processing information than younger people do. Those with high cognitive reserve also have larger neurons and less brain shrinkage with aging.

What to do? Keep your brain busy throughout your life. Even if Alzheimer's pathology gets a stranglehold on your brain, having greater cognitive reserve may enable you to cope with the damage, postponing the real tragedy of Alzheimer's—the symptoms—for years or even for your entire life.

25

BE **CONSCIENTIOUS**

**Being disciplined and responsible lessens
Alzheimer's risk**

The personality trait known as conscientiousness describes
people who are self-disciplined, goal directed, scrupulous,
purposeful, dependable, painstaking, careful, precise, orderly,
dutiful, detail oriented, and exacting. If these words describe
you, count on having a lower risk of Alzheimer's than people
with the opposite tendencies.

In fact, researchers at Rush University Medical Center in
Chicago found that elderly men and women who scored highest on tests that measure conscientiousness were about half as
likely to develop Alzheimer's twelve years later as those who
scored lowest. The most conscientious were also less apt to
experience the mild cognitive decline that precedes Alzheimer's.
Being conscientious had no effect on signs of brain pathology,
such as Alzheimer's plaques and tangles.

So what is it about being conscientious that combats
Alzheimer's? Some theories: Being conscientious helps boost

achievement and success in social, educational, and job settings, known to buck up resistance to Alzheimer's. Conscientious individuals also are more resilient and cope better with life's adversities. Thus they may be more adept at dodging trouble and chronic psychological distress, which tends to boost risk of old-age dementia.

What to do? Rejoice if you fit the conscientious profile. Keep on being responsible, honest, and hardworking to keep your brain more resistant to Alzheimer's. It's true that many conscientious people still get Alzheimer's, but evidently later in life than people who follow a less conscientious lifestyle.

KEEP **COPPER AND IRON** OUT OF
YOUR BRAIN

These two minerals can steal your memory
and promote Alzheimer's

After age fifty, excesses of copper and iron may build up in your brain, making you more vulnerable to memory impairment and Alzheimer's, according to George J. Brewer, MD, a professor emeritus of human genetics at the University of Michigan Medical School. Striking evidence of the threat is summarized in Brewer's recent report in the American Chemical Society's *Chemical Research in Toxicology.*

Simply adding copper or iron to the drinking water of lab animals increases deposits of Alzheimer's-type beta-amyloid in their brains and damages their cognitive functioning. Copper also impedes the brain's ability to get rid of amyloid plaques. Italian studies show that the more free copper there is in the blood of Alzheimer's patients, the lower their cognitive ability and the faster it deteriorates. Much research confirms that iron and copper can create toxic reactions that kill neurons and other cells.

One of the scariest findings comes from a study by prominent Alzheimer's investigator Martha Clare Morris, ScD, at Chicago's Rush University. She compared the diets and decline in cognitive functioning of thirty-seven hundred older men and women over a six-year period. In those who ingested the most copper and also ate a diet high in saturated and trans fats, cognitive functioning deteriorated rapidly, similar to the decline typical of a person who had aged *nineteen years* rather than the actual six years—that is, there was more than *three times* the expected rate of cognitive decline!

"It's frightening," says Brewer, particularly because the copper came primarily from vitamin/mineral supplements, not copper-rich foods. Brewer says that copper deficiencies are rare and that consuming copper in supplements may endanger an aging brain.

Excess iron is a well-recognized brain toxin. People with abnormally high iron levels are more prone to atherosclerosis and neurodegeneration. Alzheimer's patients often have high iron stores, and studies suggest that removing excess iron by using chelating drugs may slow the progression of dementia.

What to do? Here's advice from Brewer and other experts: Don't take iron supplements if you are a woman over age 50 (or past menopause) or an adult male, unless the iron is recommended by a health professional. Try to avoid nutritional supplements that contain copper if you eat a diet high in saturated or trans fats. Many companies offer multivitamins without iron or copper; you can find them by doing an Internet search. Eat less meat; it is rich in copper and readily absorbed heme-type iron. Try to avoid drinking water from copper pipes. Buy distilled (demineralized) water, which is cleansed of all minerals, including copper. Or use a home water-filtration system to purify tap water for drinking and cooking. Other ways to lower your iron level: donate blood, drink tea (it chelates iron), take alpha lipoic acid supplements. (See "Drink Tea," page 255, and "Consider Alpha Lipoic Acid and ALCAR," page 18.)

27

EAT **CURRY**

It has an ingredient that may chew up bad
plaque in your brain

Why does India have one of the world's lowest rates of
Alzheimer's? It's true. University of Pittsburgh research
reveals that the elderly in rural India are four times less likely
to have Alzheimer's than the elderly in Pennsylvania. One theory: curry is a staple in India, and curry powder contains the
yellow-orange spice turmeric, packed with curcumin, a compound reported to stall memory decline in both animals and
humans. One study showed that aged Asians who ate even
modest amounts of curry did better on cognitive tests. Just
eating "yellow" curries once every six months showed cognitive benefits.

Two prominent researchers, Gregory Cole, PhD, and Sally
Frautschy, PhD, at UCLA's Center for Alzheimer's Research,
who have extensively studied curcumin, say it is a potent anti-
inflammatory and antioxidant, able to slash the buildup of
Alzheimer's-inducing beta-amyloid in lab animals. Mice fed

low doses of curcumin had 40 percent fewer brain plaques than those on a normal diet.

It gets even better: aside from blocking the buildup of amyloid plaques, curcumin also nibbles away at *existing* plaques, fostering their disintegration. In short, curcumin helped rid the animal brains of established plaques, slowing cognitive decline and preventing Alzheimer's. Low doses over a longer period were more effective than high doses administered less frequently, the UCLA researchers noted.

Curcumin may be even more potent at stimulating the immune system to clear beta-amyloid from the brain when combined with vitamin D, say other UCLA investigators. (See "Don't Neglect Vitamin D," page 273.)

Curcumin also has strong anti-cancer and anti-obesity properties, as proved by research at the University of Texas M. D. Anderson Cancer Center. Specifically, curcumin can help reverse insulin resistance, high blood sugar, and high blood cholesterol, which are linked to both obesity and Alzheimer's, studies show.

Imagine if curry were a staple everywhere, as in India — we all might be less prone to cognitive decline and Alzheimer's.

What to do? Eat curry dishes frequently. One expert recommends two or three curries a week, but even an occasional curry dish is better than none. Make it a yellow curry, as yellow signifies the presence of turmeric and curcumin; green and red curries lack curcumin. And make sure the curry contains a little fat to help absorb the curcumin.

Another tack: consume the spice turmeric directly. You

can freely add it to Asian, Indian, and African dishes, such as rice, vegetables, chicken and fish stews, stir-fries, and casseroles.

You may also want to investigate curcumin supplements, sold by many companies, although curcumin is not well absorbed. For use in clinical trials, UCLA developed an "optimized" pill called Longvida that reputedly is more readily absorbed and nontoxic at a dose of under 4 grams a day. It is licensed to Verdue Science and is available online at www .longvida.com. Two 500 mg capsules a day are considered an adequate adult dose, and a higher dose might do more harm than good. However, the jury is still out on whether curcumin supplements can help prevent Alzheimer's. High doses failed in initial UCLA trials to significantly benefit people who already have the disease.

TRY THE **DASH DIET**

It can boost your scores on memory tests

The so-called DASH (Dietary Approaches to Stop Hypertension) diet, which has been hugely successful in lowering blood pressure, has an unexpected bonus: it gives your aging memory a boost, according to Heidi Wengreen, PhD, at Utah State University. She scored some 3,831 people over age sixty-five on how rigidly they stuck to the DASH diet during an eleven-year study. At the same time, the participants periodically took standardized tests to measure their rates of memory decline. Those who stuck closest to the diet had the slowest rate of cognitive decline, while the slackers who strayed most from the diet had the fastest rate of memory loss.

The diet was specifically designed by the National Institutes of Health to include foods and nutrients known to lower blood pressure. Here's the daily regimen: seven to eight servings of grains, four to five servings of fruits, four to five servings of vegetables, two to three servings of low-fat dairy, and two or fewer servings of meat. Also recommended are five servings of nuts, legumes, or seeds a week.

Researchers admit that the DASH diet is tough to follow and that nobody in the study did so 100 percent of the time. Interestingly, researchers identified four food groups most apt to benefit memory scores: vegetables, whole grains, low-fat dairy, and nuts and legumes.

British researchers have also discovered a major secret of the vegetable-loaded DASH diet's success. Vegetables, such as beets, spinach, and other leafy greens, are packed with inorganic nitrate, which is converted by the body into nitric oxide, a substance well known to relax blood vessels and lower blood pressure. In clinical trials of people with high blood pressure, the DASH diet decreased systolic blood pressure by 11 mm Hg. That's what you could expect from taking a blood pressure drug.

What to do? If you can't follow the DASH diet to the letter, do as much of it as you can. As one of the researchers said, the things you do to prevent Alzheimer's and preserve cognitive function as you age are cumulative. Every little bit can add up to a big difference. Another plus: the DASH diet plan, with tips and recipes, is free on the National Institutes of Health's website. Check it out at www.nhlbi.nih.gov/health/public/heart/hbp/dash/.

OVERCOME **DEPRESSION**

It is a risk factor for Alzheimer's, not a symptom

So you are feeling depressed, and your cognitive functioning is not what it used to be. Is this something to worry about? Yes, say experts. They know that depression is common among older people with mild cognitive impairment and Alzheimer's. But does depression bring on the disorder, or is depression a subtle early sign of the underlying pathology of Alzheimer's? Is it cause or consequence?

For ages, doctors thought depression emerged as a symptom after the disease had taken hold. Now, research suggests that the opposite is true—that depression is actually a risk factor that makes you more prone to develop Alzheimer's in the first place. In short, warding off or treating depression may save you from impending brain disaster.

For example, UCLA researchers found that depressed people with mild memory problems were more likely to end up with Alzheimer's than nondepressed people. The deeper the depression, the greater the probability.

In a French study, older women with mildly impaired mental agility who were also depressed were twice as likely to progress to Alzheimer's. Moreover, if you are depressed, you are likely to develop Alzheimer's at an earlier age, according to new University of Miami findings.

Robert S. Wilson, PhD, a neuropsychologist at the Rush Alzheimer's Disease Center in Chicago, theorizes that being depressed weakens the brain's "neural reserve," its ability to tolerate the pathology that comes with Alzheimer's. In short, he says, depression changes the brain in distinctive ways that undermine its normal resistance to the disease.

The clear message: if you're depressed, you are more apt to develop Alzheimer's, and at an earlier age, especially if you already have age-related memory problems.

What to do? Do not let depression go untreated, especially if you already notice memory problems. Drugs, including antidepressants, and other therapies, such as exercise, can make a difference. UCLA investigators also found that Aricept (donepezil), an Alzheimer's drug, significantly delayed the progression from mild memory problems to Alzheimer's in depressed persons.

30

PREVENT AND CONTROL **DIABETES**

Is Alzheimer's diabetes of the brain?

What seemed surprising a decade ago is now taken for granted: having type 2 diabetes makes you more vulnerable to Alzheimer's. Studies show it may double or triple your risk; the earlier diabetes takes hold, the higher the odds of dementia. The link is now so strong that some experts refer to Alzheimer's as "diabetes of the brain" or "type 3 diabetes."

It's still unclear exactly how diabetes converts to Alzheimer's, but here's a major clue: the two disorders have a similar genealogy of causes—obesity, high blood pressure, high cholesterol, high triglycerides, high-fat and high-sugar diets, and low physical activity, in addition to high blood sugar and dysfunctional insulin. All of these can lead to brain damage in various ways—by destroying neurons, spreading toxic seeds of dementia, and increasing inflammation and the risk of stroke. In short, diabetes can deliver a multiple whammy to the brain.

Further, subtle brain damage occurs long before overt diabetes or memory problems appear, as your body gradually loses its ability to regulate blood sugar. Among diagnosed diabetics, scores on memory tests decline as blood sugar control worsens.

The good news: controlling blood sugar helps deter dementia. Rachel A. Whitmer, PhD, at Kaiser Permanente's Division of Research in Oakland, California, has shown that the risk of Alzheimer's tumbles as blood sugar dips. Decidedly, effective blood sugar control helps prevent dementia, she says.

Suzanne Craft, PhD, a professor of psychiatry at the University of Washington School of Medicine, found that a low-saturated-fat, low-sugar diet slashed the odds of diabetics' getting Alzheimer's by normalizing insulin. On such a diet, brain levels of beta-amyloid, a hallmark of Alzheimer's, dropped about 25 percent!

Exercising and losing weight are powerful antidotes to diabetes, says a large study from Yeshiva University's Albert Einstein College of Medicine. High-risk individuals (those with high blood sugar and insulin resistance) who did moderately intense physical activity for half an hour a day five days a week and lost 7 percent of their body weight cut their diabetes odds by a remarkable 58 percent over three years. And the strategy was effective even after ten years. The over-sixty group benefited most, prompting researchers to say: it's never too late to prevent diabetes.

Other interesting ways to defeat diabetes: Sticking to the Mediterranean diet cut the odds of getting diabetes by 83 percent. Men who keep a small waist (29–34 inches versus 40–62 inches) cut their risk as much as twelve times. Eating lots of grain fiber (17 grams a day) cut diabetes odds 27 percent. Women who breast-fed reduced their diabetes risk. And diabetics who corrected periodontal problems improved blood sugar control.

What to do? Do everything possible to keep blood sugar levels low and insulin from becoming resistant so that you don't become diabetic. Critically important are a low-saturated-fat, low-sugar diet, regular exercise, and keeping weight normal. If you are diabetic, do all the same things, plus take proper medications. Although type 2 diabetes has become an epidemic, forecasting an epidemic of Alzheimer's, the evidence is clear that you can help defeat both with changes in diet and lifestyle and medical therapies. (See also "Keep Insulin Normal," page 159, and "Get a Quick Blood-Sugar Test," page 52.)

31

GET THE RIGHT **DIAGNOSIS**

If it's something else, you need to know it *now*

Too quickly assuming that an older person has Alzheimer's or just old-age memory loss can be tragic, allowing the real cause to go untreated. One example from the popular Alzheimer's Reading Room blog: "My father's internist diagnosed him with Alzheimer's disease last year (my father was then eighty) and prescribed medication that didn't seem to help him at all. It wasn't until I took my father to a neurologist that we learned he actually had a benign brain tumor."

A muddled memory, confusion, personality and mood changes, loss of balance, and other changes that mimic Alzheimer's can be caused by many treatable conditions, including a vitamin B_{12} deficiency, common in older people; a brain infection such as meningitis or encephalitis; ministrokes; a head injury; depression; side effects of medications; vascular dementia; thyroid abnormalities; even celiac disease (commonly called wheat allergy), which is increasingly found among seniors. (See "Watch Out for Celiac Disease," page 61.)

In fact, an initial diagnosis of Alzheimer's turns out to be wrong 20 to 30 percent of the time, says P. Murali Doraiswamy, MD, head of biological psychiatry at Duke University Medical Center and author of the book *The Alzheimer's Action Plan*.

Doctors, especially neurologists and geriatric specialists, have newer tests, including brain scans, that help separate Alzheimer's, a progressive brain degeneration, from temporary and correctable conditions that befuddle the aging mind. Although autopsy is still the only absolute confirmation, specialists now say they can accurately diagnose Alzheimer's about 90 percent of the time using psychoneurological exams and testing, basic blood tests, and MRI and PET brain imaging. If it's something else, you need to know *now* and get appropriate treatment before it is too late. How would you feel later if an irreversible loss could have been prevented but wasn't simply because you didn't take the time to unmask "Alzheimer's"?

What to do? If Alzheimer's is suspected, consult a neurologist, preferably a geriatric specialist, who can administer the latest tests and is experienced in recognizing brain disorders. Don't hesitate to ask your primary care physician to recommend a geriatric specialist; getting a second opinion is an acknowledged part of good medical practice. If you live near a medical college, find out if it has Alzheimer's disease specialists or a department of geriatrics. Most hospitals now also have geriatric specialists on their staffs. One of the best ways to get a prompt, reliable local referral for a medical evaluation is to contact the Alzheimer's Association at www .alz.org or 800-272-3900.

You may also be able to get a medical evaluation and/or diagnosis at one of the thirty Alzheimer's Disease Centers funded by the National Institute on Aging. For their locations and contact information, see page 299.

32

KNOW THE **EARLY SIGNS OF ALZHEIMER'S**

Surprise: memory is not the first to go

When does normal aging become abnormal? What are the very earliest recognizable behavioral signs that your brain might be turning toward Alzheimer's? The usual answer is when your memory starts giving you trouble. But memory problems are not the first clue, according to a major thirty-year collaborative study from Washington University and the University of Kansas.

A year or two before memory problems appear and three years before Alzheimer's is diagnosed, visuospatial skills begin to deteriorate, the study concluded. You may notice a decline in depth perception, says lead researcher James Galvin, MD, an associate professor of neurology at Washington University School of Medicine. You reach to pick up a glass of water and just miss it. Or you can't position your tennis racket or golf club as well to hit the ball. Parking your car seems more difficult. You misjudge the distance in walking across a street.

Doing a jigsaw puzzle or reading a map is more confusing a frustrating.

Galvin has also found that mental lapses, or "senior moments," in which you temporarily lose your train of thought, can signal developing Alzheimer's. Such episodes are called "mental fluctuations" and include excessive daytime sleepiness, staring into space for long periods, and disorganized or illogical thinking. Not everybody who has "senior moments" is on the verge of dementia, says Galvin. However, he verified that older people who frequently experience mental fluctuations are 4.6 times more likely to be diagnosed with Alzheimer's.

Losing your sense of smell can also be an early clue. Elderly people who had trouble identifying the sources of odors such as clove, lemon, pineapple, and smoke were 50 percent more likely to develop mild memory problems leading to Alzheimer's than those who had a normal sense of smell, according to research at Chicago's Rush University Medical Center.

Additionally, brain scans revealed that those with a diminished sense of smell had increased toxic beta-amyloid, even though they had no memory disturbances.

Other signs of early Alzheimer's, according to Johns Hopkins University experts, are asking the same question repeatedly; having difficulty finding the right word; misplacing belongings in odd places (like putting keys in the refrigerator); uncharacteristic behaviors, lapses in judgment, difficulty with mental arithmetic and handling money; and becoming apathetic or withdrawn.

What to do? Certainly, be on the alert for memory problems, which are a classic warning sign of Alzheimer's. (See "Recognize Memory Problems," page 189.) But also be on the lookout for pre-memory-loss signals, including a decline in visuospatial skills, mental fluctuations, and diminished sense of smell, as well as more serious signs as the disease progresses. Report concerns to your doctor, who can recommend further testing, perhaps even sophisticated brain scans. Galvin says the earlier the road signs to Alzheimer's are spotted, the more successful interventions, including lifestyle modifications and medications, are apt to be. The thrust of research is to identify the disease early, if possible, before memory is irreversibly impaired.

BE **EASYGOING AND UPBEAT**

Distress and worry bring forgetfulness and dementia

Are you easily upset, or calm and relaxed? Shy and anxious, or friendly and outgoing? Moody and apt to worry, or upbeat and seldom down? Optimistic or pessimistic? You can probably guess which personality traits please your brain more.

Yes, people with a positive, outgoing, easygoing, relaxed manner are less likely to face impaired memory and dementia as they get older. In fact, upbeat extroverts were 50 percent less likely to develop Alzheimer's than worried pessimists in a study of more than five hundred seniors at the Karolinska Institute in Sweden.

Robert S. Wilson, PhD, and colleagues at Rush University Medical Center in Chicago have discovered similar personality predictors of dementia in their research on elderly men and women participating in the long-running Religious Orders Study. Among the Catholic clergy, those who were highly prone to chronic distress and negative emotions were twice as likely to develop Alzheimer's as those with low "distress proneness." Most striking, episodic memory—the ability to recall a list of words or the details of a story—declined ten times faster among those inclined to show distress than among those more laid-back.

What's more, the researchers discovered that chronic distress (the psychological term is "neuroticism") also predicted who would develop "mild cognitive impairment," a transitional phase between normalcy and dementia. A distress-prone man or woman was about 40 percent more likely to slip into that hazardous gray area of impaired cognition than a person without that personality trait.

Especially intriguing, those prone to psychological distress and an increased risk of Alzheimer's did not have the typical brain plaques and tangles characteristic of the disease. Thus, how psychological distress makes a person more vulnerable to memory impairment and Alzheimer's symptoms is a mystery, says Rush University's David Bennett, MD, coauthor of the distress study. He notes that 90 percent of people with the clinical symptoms of Alzheimer's also have the disease's distinctive severe brain pathology. But not in cases of psychological distress. Something else is at work here that we haven't yet discovered, says Bennett.

What to do? Although Wilson notes that personality traits tend to persist throughout life, it may help to be aware that fretting, getting upset by minor frustrations, and being stressed-out and in a low mood may damage an aging brain. Try not to sweat the small stuff. Be optimistic. Take up meditation or other ways of achieving calm and serenity. Be physically active. Even a scant twenty minutes a week of any type of physical activity—including sports, housework, gardening, and walking—reduced distress and anxiety in a recent Scottish study. The more physical activity participants got, the lower their chances of psychological distress. Sports were most powerful, cutting their risk 33 percent.

Talk to your doctor about antidepressants or other medications and psychotherapy if you are chronically down. They may help prevent or alleviate cognitive problems due to distress and depression, says Wilson.

34

GET A HIGHER **EDUCATION**

It fortifies your defenses against
memory decline

Suppose two older people have similar brain changes that may lead to Alzheimer's. It's a good bet the one who stayed in school longer is less apt to actually develop symptoms of Alzheimer's. Study after study shows that the more years of formal education you have, the better your brain can withstand the pathological onslaught of Alzheimer's.

One of the most remarkable studies was done by eminent Alzheimer's researcher John C. Morris, MD, at the Washington University School of Medicine. He used PET scans to view the extent of toxic beta-amyloid deposits, signifying Alzheimer's pathology, in living brains. He also tested subjects for symptoms of Alzheimer's and noted their years of schooling. The benefits of education were startling. Among those with amyloid plaques, the more years of education, the less their memory was impaired. Those with more than sixteen years of education scored highest on cognitive tests, followed by those with thirteen to sixteen years of education, then by high school graduates or dropouts.

Higher education even trumps bad genes. German studies show that education can delay the onset of Alzheimer's in those with ApoE4 genetic susceptibility. Even among twins with identical genes, the one with more education is less apt to develop Alzheimer's symptoms.

There are several theories as to why higher education makes brains more resistant to cognitive decline and Alzheimer's. College encourages concentration, focus, reading, and other mental activities that may stimulate brain cells to build better connections. Or maybe higher education fosters better ways of compensating for failing memory as we get older. Whatever, the fact remains: people with a higher education cope better with brain damage for a longer time, say researchers, reducing the severity and delaying the symptoms of Alzheimer's.

Moreover, doing okay in school may add to brain protection. Research at the University of California, San Francisco, found that older people who said they performed "below average" in school were four times more likely to have Alzheimer's than those who said they were "average" students. However, performing "above average" did not push protection above doing just "average."

What to do? Obviously, if you can go to college and beyond, do it, because the experience is apt to enrich your life occupationally, socially, emotionally, and intellectually. Preventing Alzheimer's is an unexpected bonus. And if you didn't get a higher education when young, consider taking adult education courses, continue to learn on the job, and engage in leisure-time intellectual activities. (See "Keep Mentally Active," page 192.) All of these can add to your brain's cognitive reserve and thus your resistance to Alzheimer's.

35

AVOID **ENVIRONMENTAL TOXINS**

Everyday poisons can tilt your odds
toward Alzheimer's

Just think how much poisonous environmental stuff you inhale, ingest, and absorb over a lifetime: air pollutants, smoke, gas fumes, pesticides, cleaning agents, aluminum, lead, PCBs, iron, mercury. Many of these, such as pesticides and metals, are neurotoxins. Others trigger inflammation and oxidative damage that destroy brain tissue.

And yes, experts do say that chronic exposure to environmental toxins can increase the risks of age-related memory impairment and dementia. A recent Duke University study found that people who were exposed to occupational pesticides were 42 percent more likely to develop Alzheimer's than workers not exposed. Toxic chemicals are even more powerful than genes in bringing on dementia, say researchers at the Banner Sun Health Institute in Arizona. They recently examined brain tissue from two male identical twins, both chemical engineers who died in their late seventies. Their brains, researchers reported, "could not have looked more different." One twin, who had worked extensively with pesticides and died after a sixteen-year battle with Alzheimer's, had a brain riddled with the classic plaques and tangles of the disease. The other twin, who did not work around poisonous chemicals, died mentally sharp with a brain remarkably free of pathology. Conclusion: since the two men shared identical genes, had equal years of education, and led remarkably similar lives, pesticides were the deciding factor in which one fell victim to Alzheimer's.

Here are some other disturbing facts from a 2008 report titled "Environmental Threats to Healthy Aging," by researchers with the Greater Boston Physicians for Social Responsibility: people living in cities with severe air pollution have more Alzheimer's-type brain damage than those in cities with cleaner air. Lab rats that ingested modest amounts of aluminum had more age-related memory loss. Gardeners and farmers who used pesticides had an increased risk of mild cognitive dysfunction. Among a thousand people, those with a history of exposure to a variety of environmental toxins had an onset of cognitive decline ten years earlier than normally expected.

Brightening this dim picture is the fascinating finding that brains bolstered by more "cognitive reserve" are more resistant to damage. Among smelter workers with equally high blood levels of lead, some scored two and a half times better on tests of memory, attention, and concentration, according to neurologist Margit L. Bleecker, MD, at the Center for Occupational and Environmental Neurology in Baltimore. A critical distinguishing factor: the men less apt to be mentally impaired by toxic lead had more cognitive reserve, as indicated by higher reading scores. (See "Build 'Cognitive Reserve,'" page 77.)

What to do? Admittedly, cleaning up the environment is a public responsibility, deserving everyone's support. On a personal level, make every effort to avoid exposure to heavy metals, pesticides, and other suspected neurotoxins. Here are some suggestions from the University of California, San Francisco: Do not use pesticides. Use baits and traps instead of sprays, dusts, and bombs to control rodents and insects. Use nontoxic cleaning products. Use glass instead of plastic containers in the microwave. Wash your clothes instead of dry-cleaning them, or ask your dry cleaner to wet-clean them. The earlier and longer your exposure to environmental toxins, the greater your risk of brain problems later in life.

KNOW THE **ESTROGEN** EVIDENCE

**Whether estrogen deters dementia may
depend on when and how a woman takes it**

Sixty-eight percent of Alzheimer's patients are women. Why do more women get Alzheimer's than men? One possible reason: women live longer. But that may not be the entire story. Alzheimer's may preferentially target women because midway through life (typically at age fifty-one) they lose the protection of the hormone estrogen.

The smart solution may be to replace estrogen. That's what women routinely did until 2002, when a large National Institutes of Health study (the Women's Health Initiative) reported more heart trouble, stroke, breast cancer, and dementia in women who started taking estrogen after age sixty-five. It was a bombshell that caused millions of women to stop taking the hormone.

Leading researcher S. Mitchell Harman, MD, at the Kronos Longevity Research Institute in Phoenix, believes that forgoing estrogen may have tragic consequences. He points to extensive evidence showing that estrogen benefits an aging brain. Among other things, estrogen stimulates the growth of new neurons; strengthens dendrites and synapses, which are critical in transmitting information; raises levels of memory- and mood-regulating neurotransmitters; and improves brain circulation.

Estrogen is clearly "neuroprotective," and its rapid drop during menopause is "largely responsible for the acceleration of aging effects on cognition in women," declares Harman, who leads a major new NIH-funded study on the effects of estrogen on younger women just beginning menopause. He cites more than a dozen studies showing that estrogen improves cognition and mood and reduces memory complaints in menopausal and postmenopausal women.

However, the critical issue appears to be timing—the age at which a woman begins estrogen replacement. The original NIH study showed harm, says Harman, because the women started taking estrogen far too late, when they already had arterial and cerebral or early Alzheimer's pathology. The reintroduction of estrogen into their older bodies somehow made things worse.

It's been shown in test-tube studies that adding estrogen to brain cells already damaged by beta-amyloid (as most older brain cells are) promotes the death of neurons. In contrast, priming healthy brain cells with estrogen first and then adding beta-amyloid encourages cell survival. Thus, starting estrogen in your early fifties may benefit your brain, but starting it five to ten or even twenty years later, in your sixties or seventies, could be detrimental.

And there's more. The preferred type of estrogen replacement is estradiol, not the once-popular horse-urine-derived type used in the Women's Health Initiative study. Estradiol is plant based and identical to human estradiol, the main form of estrogen women produce before menopause. Also, an increasingly favored way to get estrogen into the body is not orally by pill but by a skin patch. Harman is testing both in his clinical trials. Natural estrogen from a patch is expected to maximize benefits and minimize side effects.

What to do? As Harman says, estrogen replacement may help save not only your brain but also your aging bones and heart. Here's his advice: Start taking estrogen immediately at the time of menopause and continue indefinitely unless your individual medical circumstances dictate otherwise. What dose? Harman says it should be low-dose transdermal estrogen (e.g., 50 mcg patch). If you are five years past menopause and haven't started estrogen, don't begin. If you started estrogen at the time of menopause or even later and then stopped using it for a period of more than five years, don't start up again. Doing so might hasten dementia and Alzheimer's as well as strokes and heart disease. Of course, always talk with your own doctor about personal issues that can help you decide whether estrogen replacement is for you.

37

ENJOY **EXERCISE**

It's like Miracle-Gro for aging brain cells

Soon after he saw the mouse brain scans, Carl Cotman, PhD, director of the Institute for Brain Aging and Dementia at the University of California, Irvine, decided to take up tennis. How could he not—or at least not start some form of vigorous exercise? The results of his mouse experiment were extraordinary. He had set up running wheels for mice to exercise on every night for a week. He was not surprised that the exercising mice were smarter than the non-exercising mice on memory and learning tests. But he was blown away by their brain scans showing that exercise had done the unthinkable: it had raised levels of the protein BDNF (brain-derived neurotropic factor) in the hippocampus, a memory-processing area that is targeted by Alzheimer's. Further, the longer the mice ran, the more BDNF their brains churned out.

This is important because BDNF acts like Miracle-Gro for

brain cells. It has been called "the master molecule of the learning process." It stimulates the growth and survival of new brain cells. Pouring BDNF over neurons in petri dishes causes cells to plump up and grow more dendrites and synapses, building new communication circuits. And that is critically important to an aging brain. If you can prevent communication breakdown from dysfunctional and dying neurons (exactly what BDNF does), you can help defeat cognitive decline and Alzheimer's, say experts.

As we age, BDNF diminishes. The lower it sinks, the lower our scores on memory tests and the faster our pace of cognitive decline. Alzheimer's patients, long before symptoms appear, have very low BDNF. So do people with mild cognitive impairment. This decline in BDNF is linked to the shrinkage of the hippocampus that drives Alzheimer's. Injecting BDNF, or molecules that mimic it, into old animals increases their rate of learning and prevents or reverses cell degeneration and death.

Cotman's trailblazing research has nailed down an easy way to get much-needed BDNF into our aging brains to fend off neuronal degeneration, memory decline, and Alzheimer's: *exercise!* And there's more. Study after study, including clinical trials, proves the extraordinary power of exercise to improve brain functioning, leading to improved cognition in older people. Scientists can see on brain scans how exercise actually increases critical blood flow to the brain and spurs neurogenesis, adding gray matter to specific cognitive-control centers.

(See "Grow a Bigger Brain," page 46.) Exercise also relieves depression and stress (reduces cortisol levels) and fights off diabetes, high blood pressure, obesity, clogged blood vessels, and insulin resistance—all associated with age-related cognitive impairment and Alzheimer's. *An important point: most studies show that aerobic exercise that leads to cardiopulmonary respiratory fitness produces more cognitive benefits than non-aerobic physical activities.* Adding resistance exercise (muscle strengthening) pushes cognitive benefits even higher.

What to do? Make exercise the cornerstone of any strategy to disassociate your brain from cognitive failure and dementia. Specifically, engage in moderate aerobic exercise ("any activity that gets your heart and lungs pumping for a sustained period of time") for an hour three times a week or a half hour five days a week. You can also do three ten-minute bouts of aerobic activity a day; it adds up to the same benefits as thirty minutes straight, say experts. Find exercise you really enjoy. Brisk walking is simple, easy, and proven. (See "Walk, Walk, Walk," page 279.) Other aerobic activities and sports expected to boost BDNF and cognitive functioning include tennis, swimming, water aerobics, calisthenics, jogging, jumping rope, and biking.

For inspiration and exercise tips and advice, explore the websites of the American College of Sports Medicine, www .acsm.org (click on "resources for general public"), and the President's Council on Physical Fitness and Sports, www .fitness.gov.

Also put these two excellent books on your reading list, both by Harvard Medical School doctors: *Spark: The Revolutionary New Science of Exercise and the Brain* by John J. Ratey (his message: "Like muscles, the brain grows with use and withers with inactivity") and *The No Sweat Exercise Plan* by Harvey B. Simon, who has developed a "cardiometabolic exercise" (CME) point system for various types of physical activity, including recreational sports, exercise workouts, walking, and around-the-house stuff, such as washing your car, vacuuming, and raking the lawn.

38

BE AN **EXTROVERT**

Your brain loves to socialize

Here's a really quirky way to measure your cognitive functioning: ask yourself how often you go to a social event. Once a day? Several times a week? Several times a month? Several times a year? Once a year? And by the way, do you have a good social support system, and how big is your network of friends and family? That's what researchers at Rush University Medical Center asked 838 older Chicagoans. The idea was to find out their level of "social engagement" and then see how it matched up with their cognitive functioning.

Let's hope you socialize frequently. The answer was unequivocal: a busy social life signified all-around better cognitive abilities in the Chicago study. People who tested higher on memory and thinking tests more often went to restaurants and sporting events; played bingo; took day trips; did unpaid community and volunteer work; visited relatives and friends; attended church or religious services; and participated in a senior center, a card-playing club, the VFW, the Knights of Columbus, or similar groups. In short, they were committed extroverts.

The mentally higher-functioning group also said they had a good social support system—friends they could count on, including "a special person who is around when I am in need."

The clear message: Being social builds a better brain. Engaging in any social activity is a pretty powerful booster of brain functioning.

What to do? If you are a natural extrovert—socially active and connected with other people—keep it up. If not, get more socially active. How can you not when you know that each social occasion and human interaction is piling up cognitive points, just like eating antioxidants or exercising? So join something, anything; go to a party; throw a party; go to a movie, a concert, or a political meeting; go out to dinner; invite people over for dinner; join a swim club, bridge club, dance club, or book discussion club. Use your imagination. "Any kind of social engagement or activity counts," says leading researcher Robert S. Wilson, PhD, of Rush University Medical Center.

39

HAVE YOUR **EYES** CHECKED

Treating vision problems may save you from Alzheimer's

If you preserve good or excellent vision as you age, your chances of developing dementia drop by an astonishing 63 percent. And if your vision is poor, just seeing an ophthalmologist for an exam and possible treatment at least once in later life cuts your dementia odds by about the same amount—64 percent. On the other hand, if you have poor vision and don't see an ophthalmologist, *your odds of getting Alzheimer's soar 950 percent!* Those are the findings of a recent study at the University of Michigan Health System.

Surprisingly, the study suggests that untreated poor vision in late life is not just a symptom of dementia but also a strong predictor of it, especially of Alzheimer's, says lead researcher Mary A. M. Rogers, PhD. Thus, treating vision problems may be an intervention strategy to delay the onset of cognitive decline and dementia. Rogers found that the likelihood of dementia dropped by 8 percent for each eye procedure done, such as removing cataracts or treating retinal problems or glaucoma. In other research, memory and learning improved significantly after cataract surgery.

Exactly how vision problems promote dementia is not totally clear. But it's logical, say researchers, that impaired vision makes it difficult to participate in mental and physical activities such as reading and exercising, as well as social activities, all believed to delay cognitive decline and Alzheimer's. Additionally, some eye diseases are tied directly to Alzheimer's pathology. For example, beta-amyloid identical to that in Alzheimer's brains can show up in the form of unusual cataracts quite unlike ordinary ones, say researchers at Harvard Medical School. British investigators at University College London found that the degree of cell death in the retina mimics that in the brain. Cells start to die ten to twenty years before the symptoms of Alzheimer's appear, they say.

Alzheimer's patients have triple the normal rate of glaucoma, a leading cause of blindness around the world. One connection, according to Francesca Cordeiro, PhD, at University College London, is that beta-amyloid damages the optic nerve just as it damages brain cells. "However, that doesn't mean that everyone with Alzheimer's will develop glaucoma or vice versa," she says. Neither disease is considered a cause of the other, but they share similar pathologies.

Swiss ophthalmologists recently discovered that many older patients who say they have trouble seeing really mean, "I can see, but I can no longer read or write." This is a sign of a visual variant of Alzheimer's disease, or VVAD, that often precedes memory complaints.

Bottom line: the signs of Alzheimer's are often reflected in the eyes, and doctors are increasingly screening patients for visual abnormalities that may indicate the early beginnings of Alzheimer's.

What to do? Be aware that your eyes reflect and influence how your brain is functioning, especially as you age. Don't tolerate poor vision. It can often be corrected, dramatically cutting your risk of dementia. See an ophthalmologist for at least one examination in late life, and have yearly screenings if possible. The doctor may also test for early visual signs of dementia. If you have trouble reading and writing, despite vision correction with lenses, see an ophthalmologist first and have a consultation with a neurologist if warranted. The point is to identify the real source of such vision problems in the earliest stages and treat them accordingly.

40

KNOW THE DANGERS OF **FAST FOODS**

They wreck the body and the brain

Since mountains of studies show that fatty, sugary fast foods promote heart disease, cancer, diabetes, obesity, and other diseases, it would be a miracle if they spared the brain. They don't. In fact, the brain is a prime organ of attack because it is so fatty and lives off glucose. It's easy, then, to believe a recent study from Sweden's renowned Karolinska Institute. It found that feeding lab animals a fast-food diet caused brain changes very similar to those in Alzheimer's patients.

The specifics: Neurobiologist Susanne Akterin, PhD, at the institute's Alzheimer's Disease Research Center, studied mice genetically modified to stand in for humans carrying the ApoE4 gene and thus highly vulnerable to Alzheimer's. For nine months, she fed them a diet high in fat, sugar, and cholesterol, chosen to mimic a fast-food diet. Postmortem examinations of their brains revealed chemical changes signifying an abnormal buildup of the protein tau. That means big trouble, because tau forms neurofibrillary "tangles," a telltale sign of Alzheimer's. She also noted that high-cholesterol foods reduced another brain substance needed for memory storage.

The message is clear: a diet of fast foods (or junk food) can put you on a faster track for Alzheimer's. When you add this to the other overwhelming evidence incriminating high-calorie, high-fat, high-sugar, high-salt fast foods in promoting obesity, insulin resistance, diabetes, high blood pressure, decreased blood flow, and stroke, you have a devastating composite picture of the damage fast foods can do.

What to do? Make a conscious decision to restrict your visits to fast-food restaurants; some experts advise no more than once a week. Or choose lower-fat, lower-calorie offerings, such as salads with olive oil or low-fat dressings. Read the nutritional information on specific fast foods, noting especially their calories, fat, and sodium. That alone may scare you off.

41

YES, YES, YES—EAT **FATTY FISH**

Fish oil is the number one fat your brain needs to prevent Alzheimer's

Your brain craves fish. Skimping on fish and its omega-3 fat dramatically ups your odds of cognitive decline and dementia, according to more than a dozen studies, says Gregory Cole, PhD, associate director of the UCLA Alzheimer's Disease Center.

"The fact is, the more fish you eat, the less likely you are to get dementia," concluded Emiliano Albanese, PhD, at King's College London, after analyzing the diets of fifteen thousand people over sixty-five in seven countries. Compared with non–fish eaters, those who ate fish a few times a week cut their odds of dementia by 20 percent, and daily fish eaters by 40 percent.

A study at Rush University Medical Center in Chicago declared that eating fish only once a week slashed the rate of cognitive decline in older people by 60 percent! It was the same as shaving *three to four years off your age*, said researchers.

Clearly, ignoring fish is hazardous to your brain. Its unique magic ingredient is omega-3 fat, made up primarily of DHA (docosahexaenoic acid) and EPA (eicosapentaenoic acid) fatty acids. It's logical, then, that high-fat fish delivers more brain protection than lean fish. For example, eating fatty fish such as salmon and tuna twice a week slashed Alzheimer's odds by 41 percent in a Tufts University study. Eating lean fish made no difference.

High blood levels of DHA predict less dementia. In a group of people ages fifty-five to eighty-eight, Tufts investigators found that those with the highest blood levels of DHA were only half as likely to develop dementia and 39 percent as likely to have Alzheimer's as those with the lowest blood DHA levels.

And more remarkable, taking pure DHA rejuvenated failing memories in older people, according to a landmark study presented at the Alzheimer's Association 2009 International Conference on Alzheimer's Disease. Older people with memory complaints who took DHA softgels (900 mg daily) for six months scored dramatically higher on a learning and memory test than those given a placebo. In fact, DHA users showed the learning and memory skills of people *three years younger,* said researchers. The DHA used in the study was provided by Martek Biosciences Corporation and was vegetarian, derived from algae. (Fish make omega-3 from eating microalgae.)

Omega-3's biochemical secrets: it stifles blood clots, extinguishes inflammatory agents, builds bigger neurons with stronger connections, destroys toxic beta-amyloid deposits and tau tangles, and slows the aging process by lengthening chromosomal cellular structures known as telomeres. (See "Take Multivitamins," page 195.)

What to do? Eat fish, primarily fatty fish such as salmon, tuna, mackerel, sardines, and herring (without cream sauce) two or three times a week or every day if you want. Canned fish has as much omega-3 as fresh. Lean fish (such as cod, whitefish, and tilapia) and shellfish are low in omega-3. Bake, broil, or steam fish. Fried fish is not a brain booster. Adding bad fats such as omega-6-rich mayonnaise, corn oil, soybean oil, or margarine diminishes the fish's benefits. (See "Beware of Omega-6 Fat," page 224.)

To be sure you get enough omega-3 fat, especially DHA, which specifically enriches brain cells, take supplements. Martek offers a 200 mg dose softgel of vegetarian DHA (www .martek.com). You can also get fish-derived capsules that combine DHA and EPA. Aim for a daily dose of 650 mg to 850 mg of omega-3 fatty acids, which will probably require a couple of 1,000 mg capsules, since not all the oil is exclusively omega-3 fatty acids. Check the label to be sure. UCLA researcher Sally Frautschy, PhD, advises taking a 200 mg capsule of algae-derived DHA and a 1,000 mg fish oil capsule (combined DHA and EPA) twice a day, once in the morning and once at night. Choose fish oil supplements that are fortified with antioxidants, such as vitamin E, to prevent rancidity. A good way to tell if a fish oil capsule is fresh: bite into it.

42

TAKE **FOLIC ACID**

This B vitamin can slow memory
decline by five years

What if you could take a pill and reverse age-related memory decline by five years? Thus, at age sixty your memory would still be as sharp as that of a fifty-five-year-old. It's not fantasy. That's exactly what happened in a Dutch study when a group of fifty- to seventy-year-olds took either 800 mcg of folic acid (a B vitamin) or a placebo (sugar pill) every day for three years. Those who took folic acid scored remarkably higher on cognitive functioning tests than those who took the placebo. In fact, the memory of the folic acid takers equaled that of someone 5.4 years younger, and their ability to process information matched that of someone 2 years younger.

In contrast the mental functioning of the sugar pill takers slid downhill as expected. This "gold standard" double-blind controlled study of 818 men and women got high praise as the first to convincingly show that folic acid slows age-related cognitive decline and possibly the onset of Alzheimer's.

Other research suggests the same. Alzheimer's patients typically have low levels of folic acid. A large study at the University of California, Irvine, showed that taking even 400 mcg of folic acid daily cut Alzheimer's risk by 55 percent in people over sixty. Feeding folic acid to old animals reduced their age-related brain damage and increased their ability to repair it, reported Mark Mattson, PhD, at the National Institute on Aging. His theory: high folic acid curbs homocysteine, a blood factor that damages brain cells' DNA. Especially revealing, Italian investigators found that people with mild cognitive impairment who also had high blood levels of folic acid were 44 percent less likely to progress to a diagnosis of dementia than those with low folic acid.

What to do? When there's the possibility of turning the clock back five years on expected memory failure, it makes superb sense to take folic acid. But there are some caveats: Be sure you are not deficient in vitamin B_{12}. High folic acid and low B_{12} are a dangerous combo and can even hasten the rate of cognitive decline. Also, if you have established heart disease or diabetes, check with your doctor before taking high doses of folic acid. There have been reports of increased kidney problems, heart attacks, and mortality risk in some people with chronic diseases who were taking high doses of folic acid—up to 2,500 mcg a day. Stick to a dose of no more than 800 mcg of folic acid a day, unless a medical professional recommends more. That dose is enough to effectively suppress Alzheimer's-related homocysteine in most people. (See "Keep Homocysteine Normal," page 144.) If you are in doubt, or have a medical problem, get the advice of a health professional on how much folic acid to take.

43

EAT A LOW-**GLYCEMIC DIET**

It protects your brain from sugar rushes

For a long time, scientists believed in two types of carbohydrates: simple and complex. Simple meant the food rapidly raised blood sugar—a prime example is plain sugar—
and complex referred to breads, grains, fruits, and vegetables,
which supposedly raised blood sugar gradually.

But that idea turned out to be wrong. The truth is more cha-
otic. Some complex carbs spike blood sugar dramatically—for
example, white potatoes and white breads are even worse than
plain sugar. The new, more accurate way of judging how carbs
affect blood sugar is by using the "glycemic index" or "glycemic
load." It is the scientific gold standard for predicting how much
and how fast a specific food raises glucose in your blood.

Not surprisingly, suppressing blood sugar spikes by eating
low-glycemic foods may help prevent diabetes and its complications, including heart disease and obesity, as well as cognitive impairment and possibly Alzheimer's. Rapid rises in blood

sugar, with resulting insulin dysfunction, can lead to mation, formation of blood clots, and detrimental changes in cholesterol and vascular structure that are not good for the brain. One Canadian study showed that type 2 diabetics did better on memory tests after eating a low-glycemic food compared to a high one (white bread). Alzheimer's is 65 percent more common in people with diabetes.

By eating a low-glycemic diet, you may delay or prevent cognitive degeneration over the years, experts suggest. You may also prevent the progression of prediabetes to full-blown diabetes.

To measure its glycemic index, each food must be tested individually for its ability to boost blood sugar; it is then assigned a number indicating its relative activity. It is not a matter of common sense. For example, you would expect prunes and dates to boost blood sugar similarly. Not so. A prune has a very low glycemic index of 29; a date has a very high one of 105.

What to do? Learn which foods are low and which are high on the glycemic index—that is, which are least apt and most apt to spike blood sugar. For a complete and regularly updated list of foods, go to www.glycemicindex.com, a website operated by the world's top experts on the subject at the University of Sydney in Australia. Avoid or restrict the foods with the high numbers, and eat more foods with the low numbers. Particularly low-glycemic foods are oats and oatmeal; legumes, including peanuts; and all vegetables, including carrots. (It's a myth that carrots spike blood sugar.) Remember, to protect your brain and the rest of your body, eating this way is not a temporary diet but a lifetime regimen.

44

GOOGLE SOMETHING

Surfing the Internet exercises your brain

It's a scientific fact: doing an Internet search can stimulate aging brains even more than reading a book. So finds Gary Small, MD, director of the UCLA Center on Aging. "Internet searching," he says, "engages complicated brain activity, which may help exercise and improve brain function."

Using MRI scans, Small measures the intensity of activity in the brains of middle-aged and older adults while they are looking up something on the Internet. He has found that activation picks up dramatically in the brains of experienced Web surfers—mainly in regions related to decision making and complex reasoning, which are *not* stimulated simply by reading. Moreover, MRIs show that savvy surfers have twice as many sparks of brain activity as novices.

Most amazing, Small found that people ages fifty-five to seventy-eight who rarely used the Internet previously were able to trigger these key centers in the brain *after only one week of surfing the Web for an hour each day.* "Searching online may be a simple form of brain exercise that might be employed to enhance cognition in older adults," he concluded.

One reason Web surfing is so demanding is that you are forced to make multiple decisions as you click, click, click to get to the ultimate information you want. Such constant decision making "engages important cognitive circuits in the brain," say researchers, giving your brain a significant workout. Mental exercise, like physical exercise, appears to strengthen your brain's resistance to mental decline and Alzheimer's. Isn't it comforting to know that this high-tech world has given us, as Small says, "a simple everyday task like searching the Web" to help keep our brains in shape?

Another way to stimulate your brain online is to play quick "brain games." For example, Posit Science (www.positscience .com) offers the 60 Second Brain Game, the Brain Speed Test, the Word List Recall, and the Farmer's Memory Challenge. Some other brain-stimulating websites noted by Small are www .brainbashers.com, www.braingle.com, www.mybraintrainer .com, www.mindbluff.com, www.neurobics.com, www.sharp brains.com, and www.syvum.com/teasers.

You can also get more complex "brain-training" programs for your computer for a few hundred dollars. These programs may work, but you should make sure they are backed up by legitimate testing and affiliated with reputable researchers, says Small. Posit Science makes the Brain Fitness Program, which has been tested on seniors in a randomized trial and found to improve scores on memory and attention tests. Other companies are doing similar scientific testing.

Nevertheless, the benefits from commercial brain training games and exercises often fall short of their "outrageous" claims, says Ronald Petersen, MD, director of the Alzheimer's Disease Research Center at the Mayo Clinic College of Medicine. He and others fear that many commercial brain-training and memory-boosting programs do not deliver what they promise, and some recent evidence confirms that.

What to do? If you don't already know how, learn to use a computer and go online to search for information, things to buy, games to play, and people to chat with. It's likely to strengthen your aging brain, as Small discovered. Still, he says, don't spend time online at the expense of socializing, walking, doing puzzles, reading (MRIs show that it, too, activates your brain), or doing other brain-building activities. (See "Keep Mentally Active," page 192, and "Do Something New," page 203.)

Look into brain-fitness-training software if it appeals to you. Check to be sure there is some solid science behind what you buy. But know that the jury is still out on how much it may benefit your brain or discourage cognitive decline or Alzheimer's. Still, if it stimulates your brain, without damaging your pocketbook, it may be worth it and better than passive, mind-numbing pursuits.

45

RAISE YOUR GOOD **HDL CHOLESTEROL**

Low HDL accelerates memory decline

I t's well known that having high good-type HDL (high-density lipoprotein) blood cholesterol protects you against heart disease. A recent study of 3,673 older people by Inserm, the French version of our National Institutes of Health, makes clear that high HDL can also save your brain.

Archana Singh-Manoux, PhD, and colleagues compared blood levels of total cholesterol, HDL cholesterol, and triglycerides with memory test scores in participants (average age fifty-five) at the beginning of the study and six years later. During those years, people with low HDL cholesterol (under 40 mg/dL) developed memory deficits at a 27 to 53 percent higher rate than those with high HDL (over 60 mg/dL). Further, short-term memory declined 60 percent faster in people with low HDL. Short-term memory loss is one of the early signs of Alzheimer's.

Why higher HDL helps you hang on to your memory is

unclear. Researchers think it may block the creation of toxic beta-amyloid, the sticky stuff that destroys brain cells, and/or act as an anti-inflammatory and antioxidant to lessen brain damage. Some research ties high HDL cholesterol to improved overall cognition, a lifetime free of dementia, and greater longevity. High HDL also boosts your odds of avoiding a stroke and of fully recovering if you suffer a mild or moderate one.

High HDLs are especially brain protective in women before and after age sixty-five, according to a major joint Swedish-American study. Women with high HDLs had better verbal ability that declined less than women with low HDLs. Incidentally, women of all ages with lower triglycerides, another type of blood fat, had dramatically better verbal and memory abilities than women with high triglycerides.

What to do? HDL cholesterol is strongly controlled by your genes, but you should try to raise it, especially if it is under 40 mg/dL. Men typically have lower HDL than women. Experts at Harvard suggest ways to ramp up HDL: exercise; drink moderate amounts of alcohol; lose weight; avoid trans fats, shown to lower HDL; eat nuts; and follow the DASH diet or the Mediterranean diet. It's also a good idea to go easy on colas. In a large Norwegian study, the more colas people of all ages drank, including diet colas, the lower their HDL. Cut back on sugar. Excess sugar, especially in processed foods, may lower good HDLs, say Emory University researchers.

You may want to ask your doctor about high doses of niacin, known to boost HDL; 1,000 to 2,000 mg a day can increase

HDL by 20 to 30 percent. Niacin is sometimes prescribed along with a statin or mixed with a statin to both lower LDL and raise HDL. *Important:* Don't risk taking high-dose niacin without medical supervision. It can cause temporary but intolerable flushing and long-term adverse effects, including gout attacks, blood-sugar elevation, and liver and muscle damage.

46

GUARD AGAINST **HEAD INJURY**

Even small blows to the head promote Alzheimer's

It's obvious that bashing your head in a car crash or bad fall can seriously harm your brain. The surprising news: so can milder blows over time, hastening the onset of Alzheimer's.

A stunning example: former National Football League players between the ages of thirty and forty-nine have *nineteen times* the rate of Alzheimer's and similar memory-related diseases as other men the same age, according to a recent University of Michigan study. In ex-players over fifty, the rate is five times higher than the national average.

Some experts call it the tip of an alarming iceberg. They worry about the long-term consequences of repeated brain blows to younger athletes. High school football players are reported to suffer forty thousand concussions a season. Boston University doctors found progressive degenerative brain disease in one eighteen-year-old high school football player who had incurred multiple concussions. It may take only three concussions to cause damage, says one expert.

Professional boxers may end up punch-drunk. Amateur boxers, although they wear helmets and are rarely knocked out, display brain injuries that predict cognitive decline, say Swedish investigators. Logically, hockey, rugby, and soccer players, wrestlers, and anybody who plays a contact sport is in jeopardy.

Still, what's "blatantly obvious" to brain researchers is not widely known, warns Samuel Gandy, MD, an Alzheimer's disease research professor at Mount Sinai School of Medicine: *multiple concussions dramatically increase the risk of neurological degeneration years later.*

For that matter, banging your head at any age may increase your susceptibility to Alzheimer's. A Columbia University analysis found Alzheimer's nearly four times more common in elderly people who had suffered a head injury. Older people who severely injured their heads in accidental falls were two and a half times more apt to have cognitive decline or dementia five years later, according to a Finnish study.

A further concern is that those who carry the ApoE4 gene have a particularly high risk of dementia after brain trauma. It is so significant that one expert suggests screening athletes for ApoE4. The idea is to identify the most vulnerable so they can decide whether to incur the higher risk of long-term neurological consequences that come with contact sports.

What to do? Everything possible to protect your brain. Buckle your seat belt. Always wear a helmet in sports where the head is exposed and when riding a bicycle, motorbike, or motorcycle. It won't provide 100 percent protection but may lessen the brain damage from a fall. Fall-proof your house. Be especially careful if you carry the extra risk of ApoE4. (See "Know About the ApoE4 Gene," page 32.) Tiny blows today may turn into serious dementia later in life.

47

BE GOOD TO YOUR **HEART**

What destroys your heart destroys your memory

The good things you do for your heart are reflected in your brain. Scientists now recognize that the destroyers of your blood vessels and heart also wreck your brain.

The same bad saturated fats that clog arteries weaken the blood-brain barrier, allowing toxic beta-amyloid to plant the seeds of Alzheimer's in brain cells, says Australian research. Plaque buildup in your carotid (neck) arteries signals a faster rate of cognitive decline and memory loss, warn University of Maryland researchers. If you have peripheral artery disease (PAD), your risk of Alzheimer's goes up. Atrial fibrillation, a form of abnormal heart rhythm, as well as cerebral artery disease, makes you more vulnerable to strokes. A-fib alone doubles your risk of Alzheimer's and triples your risk of vascular dementia. Reduced blood flow and clots kill both heart muscle and brain mass. High inflammation in arteries, high blood pressure, high homocysteine, high LDL (bad) cholesterol, and low HDL (good) cholesterol all ramp up your odds of heart disease and dementia. A sedentary lifestyle damages both your heart and brain. So does a potbelly. And on and on...

The strong message: look after your heart if you want to grow old with your memory intact. Neurologist Charles DeCarli, MD, at the University of California, Davis, School of Medicine, says that the things you do to keep your heart healthy may be even more important for your brain. "Some heart damage can be repaired surgically, but not brain damage," he points out. "A memory lost is never recovered."

Jack de la Torre, MD, at the Center for Alzheimer's Research at Banner Sun Health Research Institute in Arizona, suggests that all healthy middle-aged individuals be screened by three simple, noninvasive tests—carotid artery ultrasound, echocardiogram, and ankle-brachial index—to detect and treat Alzheimer's cardio risk factors long before cognitive symptoms appear. That systematic strategy alone, he says, could delay or prevent countless cases of cognitive impairment, dementia, and Alzheimer's.

What to do? Go for regular and thorough cardiovascular checkups. Ask for sophisticated blood tests that measure levels of LDL and HDL cholesterol; measure homocysteine and C-reactive protein (CRP), a marker of inflammation; and show ApoE factors, if you want to know your genetic vulnerability to Alzheimer's. Take de la Torre's advice and get these additional tests: a Doppler ultrasound to detect blockages of narrow places that restrict blood flow, an ankle-brachial index test for peripheral artery disease, and an echocardiogram to detect abnormalities that may restrict blood flow to the brain. (See "Check Out Your Ankle," page 24.) Exercise, follow both the Mediterranean and a low-glycemic-index diet, and take heart medications if needed. A smarter brain is a great bonus for taking good care of your heart.

KEEP **HOMOCYSTEINE** NORMAL

This toxin in your arteries also
targets your brain

A high blood level of an amino acid called homocysteine is typically associated with heart disease. It also predicts age-related memory loss, stroke, dementia, and Alzheimer's, say a string of studies.

As homocysteine goes up, so does your likelihood of dementia, according to an analysis of the large Framingham Heart Study. The odds of Alzheimer's nearly doubled in older people with high blood homocysteine levels, greater than 14 micromoles per liter (μmol/L).

In recent Swedish research at the University of Gothenburg, women with the highest homocysteine in middle age, compared to those with the lowest, were three times more likely to have a stroke and two and a half times more likely to develop Alzheimer's two to three decades later. High homocysteine also raises your odds of age-related cognitive impairment, which precedes dementia, by 240 percent, say University of Michigan researchers. Having both high homocysteine and the ApoE4 Alzheimer's gene damages cognitive functioning more than either hazard alone, University of Maine researchers discovered. In short, homocysteine magnifies the risk of bad genes; thus it is especially imperative for ApoE4 carriers to control homocysteine.

How homocysteine might lead to brain damage is unclear, but based on animal studies, scientists believe that high homocysteine somehow facilitates a buildup of toxic beta-amyloid and tau in brain cells, the two hallmarks of Alzheimer's.

Now the good news: zapping homocysteine is fairly easy. People with high homocysteine typically are deficient in B vitamins. Strikingly, in the Framingham Heart Study, those with the lowest blood levels of B vitamins, compared to those with the highest, were *six times* more apt to have high homocysteine. So it follows that taking B vitamins can reduce homocysteine and also the risk of cognitive decline and Alzheimer's. But it's still unproven whether the act of getting homocysteine down keeps you safe from dementia. Regardless, high homocysteine spells cognitive danger ahead and keeping it normal makes a lot of preventive sense.

What to do? Ask your doctor about a simple, inexpensive test to find out how high your homocysteine is. It is often done at the same time blood is drawn for cholesterol testing. Standard guidelines say from 5 to 15 μmol/L of homocysteine is normal.

However, studies suggest that lower is far safer. A daily regimen of three B vitamins — folic acid (800 mcg), B_{12} (1,000 mcg), and B_6 (25 mg) — is usually enough to lower homocysteine and correct deficiencies of these vitamins in most older people. (See "Take Folic Acid," page 127.)

49

AVOID **INACTIVITY**

Being a couch potato makes you a magnet
for Alzheimer's

Unquestionably, being physically inactive makes you a more attractive target for memory loss and Alzheimer's. Generally, the more sedentary you are, the faster your cognitive decline.

University of California, San Francisco, researchers found that older adults who were sedentary (did not exercise at all) had the worst cognitive functioning at the start of a seven-year study and the steepest rates of decline throughout the study. In fact, the couch potatoes' cognitive test scores dropped 55 percent more than those of participants who maintained a higher activity level (at least 150 minutes of walking a week). Mental skills also slipped faster in people who consistently did less physical activity during the seven-year study.

The main message, says lead researcher Deborah E. Barnes, PhD: even if you've stopped exercising, start again. If you are active, maintain or increase your exercise levels. "The worst thing is to stay sedentary."

Studies suggest that staying physically active reduces the risk of developing Alzheimer's by up to 40 percent. Even doing *some* physical activity, compared with none, "has a protective effect against Alzheimer's," says prominent Alzheimer's authority Nikolaos Scarmeas, MD, at Columbia University College of Physicians and Surgeons. He found that older people who did as little as fifty minutes a week of moderate activity, such as bicycling, swimming, hiking, or playing tennis, were 25 percent less likely to develop Alzheimer's than those who did none.

A recent Mayo Clinic study found that getting any moderate exercise, no matter how often, in midlife or late life cuts your odds of mild cognitive impairment by more than 30 percent.

Why is physical inactivity so hard on the brain? For one reason, it leads to visceral, or belly, fat, which triggers persistent low-grade inflammation, incriminated as a promoter of Alzheimer's, say Danish researchers. In contrast, they note that physical activity, involving contractions of skeletal muscles, releases hormone-like anti-inflammatory agents, fending off brain damage.

Additionally, physically inactive people, as shown on MRIs, have less blood flow in the brain and more brain shrinkage as they age, notably in the hippocampus, an area central to memory and learning.

What to do? Get up and move. Do what you can; every bit of activity helps. It need not be vigorous and intense; moderate aerobic exercise gets most experts' vote as the most likely path to significant brain benefits. That means aiming for thirty minutes of moderate exercise or fifteen minutes of intense exercise a day. But know that getting off the couch and moving at any pace, no matter how slow, is your first act in saving your aging brain. You can always rev it up as you go.

Another simple way to overcome inactivity is to wear a pedometer (a step counter) and gradually increase how many steps you take daily. Here's an activity gauge, according to University of Arizona exercise specialists: under 5,000 daily steps is "sedentary"; 5,000–7,499 daily steps, "low active"; 7,500–9,999 daily steps, "somewhat active"; more than 10,000 daily steps, "active"; and more than 12,500 daily steps, "highly active." (See "Be a Busy Body," page 54, "Build Strong Muscles," page 198, and "Walk, Walk, Walk," page 279.)

50

TRY TO KEEP **INFECTIONS** AWAY

Pathogens in the brain may be an underlying cause of Alzheimer's

Is it possible that infections could trigger Alzheimer's? Some scientists believe so. The idea is very controversial and gaining renewed attention. Recently, the *Journal of Alzheimer's Disease* devoted a special issue to emerging evidence linking Alzheimer's to common microorganisms that cause cold sores, gastric ulcers, Lyme disease, pneumonia, and even the flu.

Scientists know that infectious agents hang out in Alzheimer's brains. Leading researcher Brian Balin, PhD, at the Philadelphia College of Osteopathic Medicine, discovered *Chlamydia pneumoniae* bacteria in 90 percent of brain samples from deceased Alzheimer's patients, compared to only 5 percent of samples from normal brains. The implications are enormous, since this pathogen is one cause of community-acquired pneumonia, a common infection, especially in people over age sixty-five.

Remarkably, after Balin let normal non-Alzheimer's-prone

mice sniff the *C. pneumoniae* bacteria, their brains also developed toxic amyloid deposits—rare even in such aged mice. This proves, he says, that the infectious agent can initiate Alzheimer's pathology, causing the disease.

Herpes simplex virus type 1 (a cause of cold sores) is also a prime suspect. The DNA of the virus is three times more apt to show up in the plaques of Alzheimer's brains than in normal brains, says Ruth Itzhaki, PhD, at the University of Manchester in England. She calls the virus "a major cause of amyloid plaques" and estimates that the cold sore virus could cause about 60 percent of all Alzheimer's cases.

Another potential culprit: *Helicobacter pylori* bacteria, which cause gastric and peptic ulcers. In a Greek study, Alzheimer's patients were nearly twice as likely to have *H. pylori* infections as normal patients.

There's also evidence that a common influenza virus may settle in your brain, leading to neurodegenerative damage. And Canadian research has found the Lyme disease infection spirochete (*Borrelia burgdorferi*) residing in Alzheimer's brain tissue alongside amyloid plaques.

Here's the theory, explains Balin: Various microbes, inhaled or taken into the blood, enter the brain, causing an infection that becomes chronic, perhaps lingering for years undetected. The infection triggers toxic beta-amyloid production and encourages neuronal destruction precisely in the areas of the brain governing memory and cognition. Thus the infection is the underlying cause of the plaque that triggers Alzheimer's.

Especially unsettling: some pathogens, such as *C. pneumoniae*, may float in the communal air and be quickly inhaled directly into the brain. That raises this intriguing question: if Alzheimer's is airborne, might it even be contagious? "Possibly," says Balin, although he points out that many other factors would influence whether it actually ends up as Alzheimer's.

There is growing evidence that beta-amyloid brain buildup is tied to infection. As we age, low-grade infections may trigger the immune system to produce beta-amyloid as a kind of "antibiotic" to defend brain cells, says Rudolph Tanzi, PhD, at Massachusetts General Hospital's Institute for Neurodegenerative Disease. Indeed, Tanzi has demonstrated that beta-amyloid inhibits the growth of eight organisms, including *Candida albicans*, listeria, staphylococcus, and streptococcus. The theory: a little beta-amyloid initially may be protective, but lots of it over a long period goes awry and becomes lethal to brain cells.

What to do? Take precautions to avoid infections. Get appropriate vaccinations. In a Canadian study of people over age sixty-five, those who said they had been vaccinated against diphtheria or tetanus, poliomyelitis, and influenza were as much as 60 percent less apt to develop Alzheimer's. Taking antibiotics and antiviral agents when needed may also benefit your brain. (See "Don't Shy Away from Antibiotics," page 26.) Keep alert for emerging evidence on this intriguing potential risk factor.

51

FIGHT **INFLAMMATION**

That fire in your brain promotes dementia

Not long ago, scientists thought it was impossible for inflammation to occur in brain tissue. They were wrong. Low-level inflammation can persist in your brain, destroying neurons and making you a more vulnerable target for memory loss and Alzheimer's, says prominent researcher Joseph Rogers, PhD, at the Banner Sun Health Research Institute in Arizona, an Alzheimer's Disease Center of the National Institute on Aging.

Although why such chronic inflammation settles in your brain is not entirely understood, its devastation is a terrible sight to see under a microscope, says Rogers. Essentially, it is a normal immune system response gone awry, he explains. Immune scavenger cells, called microglia, view toxic beta-amyloid (present in normal as well as diseased brains) as a "foreign invader" and launch fierce attacks to remove it. In the process, the microglia overreach and inadvertently destroy millions of healthy bystander brain cells essential for memory and thinking. Over time, this continual low-grade immune activation creates a mess of dead and dysfunctional brain cells, promoting Alzheimer's, says Rogers.

How can you tell if brain inflammation may be a problem? You can get an indirect answer through a blood test that measures inflammatory agents. At least ten studies show that high blood concentrations of inflammation markers, such as C-reactive protein (CRP), are associated with a higher risk of dementia and memory impairment. In one large twenty-five-year study, people with the highest CRP levels, compared to those with the lowest, were nearly three times as likely to develop dementia. Recent Mayo Clinic research found a 40 percent higher risk of mild cognitive impairment in those with high levels of blood inflammation. No question, say experts: inflammation is a prime enemy of the aging brain.

What to do? Everything that may help tame inflammation. For one thing, have a CRP blood test to find out your inflammation status. To fight inflammation, stay physically active, aiming for thirty to forty-five minutes a day of brisk walking. Eat fatty fish and/or take fish oil supplements; omega-3 fat in fish is extremely anti-inflammatory. Restrict highly inflammatory saturated fats, trans fats, and omega-6 fat. Eat a Mediterranean diet. Shrink your waist size; visceral, or belly, fat is pro-inflammatory. Seek out nutrients and antioxidants that are anti-inflammatory—for example, curcumin in curry, vitamin C, vitamin E, and alpha lipoic acid. Statins have strong anti-inflammatory properties, which some experts think is a primary reason they may work against heart disease, although studies do not find statins effective in preventing Alzheimer's. (See "Investigate Statins," page 242.)

FIND GOOD **INFORMATION**

Keeping up on reliable scientific research can help you ward off dementia

Searching for ways to prevent, delay, and slow down the onset and progression of Alzheimer's (hopefully for a lifetime) is now a high priority among many researchers, and they regularly come up with new strategies to reduce your risk. Thus, you need to stay on top of these findings. In the glut of Internet information and misinformation, knowing where to look for the latest *scientifically reliable research and advice* is good brain protection.

What to do? Here are some of the leading sources of top-quality information you can count on to both engage your brain and help save it:

The <u>National Institute on Aging,</u> under the umbrella of the National Institutes of Health, funds most of the research on Alzheimer's and dementia in the United States. Its huge website can keep you up-to-date about ongoing studies, diagnostic advances, and the impact of various strategies, such as exercise, diet, and lifestyle, on your aging brain. Go to www.nia .nih.gov.

The Alzheimer Research Forum is a very lively and well-written website that posts comments from both leading authorities on Alzheimer's and the general public. It reports the latest research, carries discussions among experts, and gives full exposure to innovative, controversial, and offbeat theories and ideas. It's the place to go to find out the complete range of what top researchers in the field are thinking and doing. Go to www .alzforum.org.

Alzheimer's Disease Centers, funded by the National Institute on Aging, are located at major medical institutions around the country. They carry out the most important and cutting-edge research on preventing and curing Alzheimer's. They also offer information, diagnosis, medical management, and opportunities for participating in clinical trials. They are extremely reliable sources of information. For a listing of thirty centers with websites and phone numbers, see the appendix, page 299.

The Alzheimer's Association is a national nonprofit organization with local chapters and a website offering extensive information on the disease. Be sure to check out its excellent interactive tour of the brain, which shows how the brain works and how Alzheimer's destroys it. Go to www.alz.org. For the brain tour, click on "Alzheimer's Disease," then "Brain Tour." It's available in several different languages. For medical referrels and other support, call 800-272-3900.

Pub Med, operated by the National Library of Medicine at

the National Institutes of Health, is an online service that gives you access to virtually all scientifically published studies worldwide (more than nineteen million) on various diseases and health problems, including Alzheimer's, dementia, cognitive decline, and mild cognitive impairment. You can search by subject, author's name, journal title, or article title. The abstract (summary) is free, although you may have to pay a fee to download the entire article. This is the place to go if you want to check the scientific validity of something you have read on the Internet or in a publication or have heard on radio or TV. If the technical language is confusing, go to the end of the abstract or paper for the "conclusions" or "discussion" to find the major points. Go to www.pubmed.gov.

53

KEEP **INSULIN** NORMAL

Abnormal and weak insulin is a serious brain threat

If your insulin gets out of whack, your brain is in deep trouble. Insulin is the hormone that prods cells to absorb glucose from food, providing energy to carry on life processes. Insulin is surprisingly powerful in your brain, says leading Alzheimer's researcher Suzanne Craft, PhD, at the University of Washington School of Medicine. The hormone facilitates memory formation and blocks the activity of toxic beta-amyloid, which is intent on destroying your brain.

Normally, insulin is diligent. But it can lose the strength to carry on, precipitating catastrophic cognitive problems and a possible takeover of your brain by diabetes and dementia. This can happen when cells become insensitive or resistant to insulin's advances. When cells refuse to accept and process glucose, it spills over into intercellular spaces. The pancreas then pours out more insulin in a misguided attempt to correct the glucose overload. Soon your blood is awash in unprocessed sugar and useless insulin. This condition is called "insulin resistance." It is a primary underlying cause of diabetes, says Craft, as well as a contributor to brain inflammation, microvascular disease, and the amyloid plaques and tau tangles that promote strokes, memory impairment, and Alzheimer's.

The good news: insulin resistance is preventable and treatable. Craft can induce insulin resistance by having people eat a high-saturated-fat, high-sugar diet for only four weeks! She can reverse it in the next four weeks by switching them to a low-saturated-fat, low-sugar diet. She explains that saturated fat and sugar are a vicious combo: sugar causes insulin and blood glucose to spike, and saturated fat keeps them abnormally elevated for a very long time. More alarming, Craft has documented that people on high-fat diets have more beta-amyloid in their central nervous systems—but it decreases within a month of switching to a low-fat diet.

Exercise, notably aerobic exercise, is also a potent treatment for insulin resistance. "It is dramatic and immediate," says Craft. "One thirty-minute bout of aerobic exercise improves your insulin function for twenty-four hours." Best of all: the right diet and exercise together produce better control than either alone.

What to do? Right now there are no simple, reliable tests for insulin resistance, but if your blood sugar tests high or if you have been diagnosed with diabetes or prediabetes, it's a good bet you have insulin resistance. One out of four Americans over age sixty do, and most don't know it.

Normalizing insulin may be the biggest favor you can do for your aging brain. Try these strategies to keep insulin normal: Lose weight. Get off the saturated fat and sugar. Eat foods that are low on the glycemic index, which has been shown to reverse insulin resistance. Do aerobic exercise every day if you can, or at least three times a week. Eat cinnamon and vinegar to suppress the blood glucose spikes that lead to high insulin levels. (See "Go Crazy for Cinnamon," page 71, and "Put Vinegar in Everything," page 269.)

54

HAVE AN INTERESTING **JOB**

Work that excites your brain makes it stronger

Sure, a good salary and a high-status job may make you happy. But your brain thrives on work that makes you think. People who keep learning on the job have a lower risk of dementia, including Alzheimer's, according to researcher Guy Potter, PhD, an assistant professor of psychiatry at Duke University Medical Center.

In his study of identical male twins, those with jobs that demanded higher reasoning, language, and math skills were less prone to Alzheimer's. Not surprisingly, that group included doctors, lawyers, engineers, professors, authors, architects, and accountants. "But it is not only white-collar professionals who use their intellect," Potter points out. Those in lower-status jobs who take regular vocational training and education courses needed to move up the ladder also reduce their risk of dementia.

Similarly, Kathleen Smyth, PhD, at Case Western Reserve

University, found that getting stuck in a mentally undemanding job during midlife boosted the risk of Alzheimer's, whereas moving on to a more mentally challenging job cut the risk. And if you missed out on a higher education, having a stimulating lifetime occupation can help make up for it in protecting against Alzheimer's, say researchers.

One of the most fascinating studies, showing that you don't need a fancy workplace or job title to stimulate your brain, involved London taxi drivers. Using brain imaging, Eleanor A. Maguire, PhD, a researcher at University College London, documented that taxi drivers, who must memorize and navigate London's complex routes of winding streets and landmarks to qualify for a license, actually grew bigger brain cells. They clearly had more gray matter in the hippocampus, a memory-forming region of the brain, than ordinary automobile drivers, and the more years they drove a taxi, the more gray matter they accumulated. In contrast, London bus drivers, who automatically follow a set route, did not show increased gray matter. Maguire concluded that the demanding mental expertise of driving a London taxi actually caused the enlargement of nerve cells in the relevant region of brain anatomy. Interestingly, after the taxi drivers retired, the amount of gray matter in their hippocampi returned to normal in a few years.

What to do? Choose an occupation where you have to use your mind. Participate in ongoing opportunities for learning and advancement on the job. If possible, avoid jobs that are boring and mentally unchallenging. The key is ongoing learning, say researchers. On the other hand, as Smyth notes, "not everybody can be an astrophysicist." She says you can help counteract the downside of a less stimulating job by keeping your mind active outside of work. She advises "novelty-seeking" activities and taking educational courses. (See "Do Something New," page 203.)

55

DRINK **JUICES** OF ALL KINDS

A glass every day or two slashes your odds of getting Alzheimer's

It's easy to get up in the morning and have a glass of juice. It's also startling how much that simple act can slash your chances of Alzheimer's. Compelling research from the Vanderbilt University School of Medicine in Nashville shows that the risk of Alzheimer's plummeted 76 percent in people who drank fruit or vegetable juice more than three times a week, compared to those who drank juice less than once a week. Drinking juice once or twice a week cut Alzheimer's odds by 16 percent.

Experts know that deeply colored juices, such as Concord (purple) grape juice, pomegranate juice, and blueberry juice perform miracles in lab animal brains. When given pomegranate juice, mice genetically altered to get Alzheimer's had only half as much brain buildup of beta-amyloid plaques and lower odds of Alzheimer's than mice drinking plain water, according to research at Loma Linda University in California.

On maze tests, pomegranate-juice-drinking mice were much smarter, faster, and more efficient than water-drinking mice.

Fascinating research by James Joseph, PhD, at Tufts University and Robert Krikorian, PhD, at the University of Cincinnati showed that drinking Concord grape juice or commercial blueberry juice improved short-term and verbal memory in older people with early memory loss and a high risk of Alzheimer's. Those who drank about two glasses of 100 percent Concord grape juice a day for twelve weeks were better able to memorize lists than those who got a placebo drink.

Similarly, in another test, seniors with mild cognitive impairment who drank commercially available wild blueberry juice for twelve weeks improved by 40 percent on one memory function test and by 20 percent on a word list recall test. The subjects drank 1¾ to 2½ cups of blueberry juice daily, depending on their body weight.

Joseph and Krikorian credit the extremely high concentrations of antioxidants (polyphenols) in the dark purple and blue juices. They note that red and white grape juices are much lower in antioxidants and less effective as cognitive boosters.

Many fruit and vegetable juices have not been closely scrutinized for their brain-protecting potential, so it is impossible to be sure which are most potent. Some research suggests that tomato juice, high in the antioxidant lycopene, may protect aging brains. Apple juice, on the other hand, is lower in overall antioxidant power, but it has other tricks that make it a good bet against Alzheimer's. (See "Drink Apple Juice," page

35.) Orange juice has newly discovered anti-inflammatory properties.

What to do? What's to lose? Why not make it a habit to drink a glass of juice every day? It's hardly a hazardous gamble, since fruits and vegetables of all kinds help save you from countless disorders and diseases. Alzheimer's and premature memory loss are just for starters. And mix it up. It may be smart to drink more of the deep-colored, brain-proven juices, such as grape, pomegranate, and blueberry juice, but don't forget orange and grapefruit, pineapple, mango, cherry, prune, and all the rest. They, too, are apt to have brain benefits. Be sure to drink only 100 percent fruit or vegetable juices, not "fruit drinks." Look for "no sugar added" on the label. If you can't find wild blueberry juice locally, the Van Dyk's brand used in the Tufts–University of Cincinnati studies is available at www .vandykblueberries.ca.

56

LEARN TO LOVE **LANGUAGE**

Linguistic skills build bigger, smarter, stronger brains

The ability to write about sophisticated ideas with a great deal of clarity and complexity early in life makes you less likely to have Alzheimer's later in life. And those early linguistic skills triumph even if you develop severe brain pathology that fits a diagnosis of Alzheimer's. That is the fascinating conclusion of research on more than six hundred elderly Catholic women in the United States who participated in the so-called Nun Study.

Leading researcher Suzanne Tyas, PhD, at the University of Waterloo in Ontario, looked at essays handwritten by nuns at the time they entered the convent in their late teens or early twenties. The autobiographical essays were scored for their "density of ideas" and "grammatical complexity." The purpose was to compare the literary quality of the early writing with each nun's cognitive state in old age, while taking into consideration the extent of her brain pathology.

The striking finding: clearly, nuns with superior early literary abilities were more likely to be free of dementia in their seventies, eighties, and nineties than those who began with lesser language skills. Of 180 women studied, about one third had brain damage meriting a diagnosis of Alzheimer's. Yet only half of those with brain damage ever showed symptoms of dementia during their lives. Most revealing: women who scored in the top three quarters for linguistic skills, compared with those in the bottom quarter, were seven to eight times more apt to be free of dementia symptoms despite having brain damage that indicated Alzheimer's pathology.

Tyas suggests that "linguistic ability may be one of those early-life characteristics that reflects reserve capacity, helping us resist the clinical expression of Alzheimer's." In short, a more literate brain when young may counter an Alzheimer's takeover in old age.

Being bilingual from childhood also delays the onset of dementia by four years, says a Canadian study by Ellen Bialystok, PhD, a professor of psychology at York University. Dementia occurred at the average age of 75.5 years in fluent speakers of two languages, compared to age 71.4 years in monolingual speakers. Israeli researchers found that the more languages an older person spoke, the better their cognitive state. The theory: handling more than one language constantly exercises and strengthens the brain.

What to do? If you're young, be inspired toward a literate life. If you are older, continue to read widely and write extensively to express your thoughts. Think about learning languages other than your native one. Expose children to different languages. Take writing courses. Research shows that continuing to acquire linguistic skills stimulates your brain no matter what your age. "The notion of recommending language acquisition as a kind of mental exercise that might lower one's risk for Alzheimer's follows logically," says Samuel Gandy, MD, professor of Alzheimer's disease research at the Mount Sinai School of Medicine in New York.

57

AVOID A **LEPTIN DEFICIENCY**

High levels of the "hunger hormone" cut the risk of Alzheimer's

An appetite-suppressing hormone that tells your brain to stop eating because you are full may also stop the brain damage leading to Alzheimer's. A blockbuster study by researchers at Boston University found that you are four times less likely to develop Alzheimer's if you have high blood levels of the "hunger" hormone, leptin, compared to low levels.

Wolfgang Lieb, MD, and colleagues measured leptin in a large group of elderly men and women, then followed them for twelve years to see who developed Alzheimer's. The risk was 25 percent in those with the lowest leptin levels and 6 percent in those with the highest—a fourfold difference, which leptin researcher J. Wesson Ashford, MD, at Stanford University, said is "a huge thing," about as risky as having the ApoE4 gene. "It means that if you were to take people with low leptin levels and convert them to a high leptin level, you could delay Alzheimer's by ten years," says Ashford.

Moreover, MRI scans showed that the seniors with higher leptin levels had more brain volume in the hippocampus, a key memory center, than those with lower levels. However, high leptin did not cut dementia risk in obese individuals, probably because they tend to develop resistance to it, just as many people become resistant to the hormone insulin. Leptin is secreted by fat cells and implicated in obesity and diabetes.

In other research, leptin also seemed to slow cognitive decline. Older people with high blood levels of leptin were 34 percent less apt to experience cognitive decline than those with low leptin, according to a study of 2,871 individuals by Karen Holden, MD, at the University of California, San Francisco.

Leptin's possible role in Alzheimer's is no surprise to many neuroscientists. In animals, leptin improves memory and reduces brain levels of amyloid and tau, both hallmarks of Alzheimer's.

What to do? Manipulating the hormone leptin is tricky and not totally understood, but the same things that fight diabetes appear to improve leptin. Most important, say experts, is habitual aerobic exercise; it makes leptin more sensitive. You should also cut sugar intake, especially added fructose, as in high-fructose corn syrup; a high-fructose diet can induce leptin resistance. (Fructose naturally occurring in fruit is probably not a danger.) Eat fatty fish and take fish oil; omega-3 fat improves leptin. Eat less animal fat and trans fat; switching lab animals from a high-fat to a low-fat diet normalized leptin. Control blood sugar and obesity; both are detrimental to leptin.

58

DON'T BE **LONELY**

It doubles your odds of Alzheimer's

Being lonely is different from being alone, says Robert S. Wilson, PhD, a Rush University psychologist and lead author of a study on loneliness and the risk of Alzheimer's. "Loneliness is not just social isolation; it is emotional isolation," he says. "It is feeling alone, not just being alone."

To measure loneliness, Wilson and colleagues asked eight hundred older people how much they agreed with a series of statements, including "I experience a general sense of emptiness," "I miss having people around," "I feel like I don't have enough friends," "I often feel abandoned," and "I miss having a really good friend."

Loneliness emerged as a prime predictor of Alzheimer's. People with the highest loneliness scores were twice as apt to develop Alzheimer's as those with the lowest. Further, the loneliest had the most rapid declines in various types of memory and cognitive functioning over a four-year period.

Why loneliness is so hard on the brain is unclear. Wilson speculates it may somehow "compromise" neural systems. For example, in animals subjected to social isolation, brain cells shrink in critical memory centers, resulting in impaired memory. His study also suggests that for some lonely people, being *satisfied* with current social interactions may count more in delaying Alzheimer's than just having a large social circle. Such people say they still feel lonely even though they appear to have friends and are socially active.

Who's most vulnerable? Not surprisingly, older people who live alone and have experienced the death of a spouse or an intimate friend, says a recent Australian study. This research also found less loneliness among older people who interacted with family (especially children and grandchildren), sought out younger friends, arranged food-related gatherings, had pets, and spent time gardening and reading.

What to do? It's not easy, since loneliness strikes at various ages and may be more of a personality trait than the result of circumstances, says Wilson. He suggests therapy and possibly antidepressants (loneliness is tied to depression) to help stop cognitive damage, preferably before it becomes severe. Also, you should avoid social isolation; it worsens loneliness. If you know older people who are lonely, reach out to them. Any bit of social interaction may mean a lot. Don't let a brain die of loneliness.

59

EMBRACE **MARRIAGE**

Staying coupled makes your brain happier

Try this unorthodox test for predicting Alzheimer's: look at your ring finger (the one next to the pinky) on your left hand. That's right: your marital status is a mega clue, according to a large study from Sweden and Finland. Being married or living with a significant other keeps Alzheimer's away. Living alone makes you much more vulnerable, especially if you're a woman.

The specifics: Academic researchers gathered personal information on about fifteen hundred middle-aged individuals and then checked on them twenty-one years later for signs of dementia. The correlation with emotional coupling was striking. Having a partner in midlife (around age fifty) cut the risk of being cognitively impaired after age sixty-five in *half.* In contrast, middle-aged singles (the divorced, widows, widowers, and never-marrieds) were two to three times more apt to have dementia in late life than members of a couple.

Widows going it alone had six times the risk of Alzheimer's. Most vulnerable of all were widows living solo who also carried the ApoE4 genetic risk factor for Alzheimer's. Their risk of Alzheimer's shot up fourteen times over that of cohabitating couples not genetically prone to the disease.

How to explain it? Admittedly, it's amazing that the social and emotional ties of marriage and committed coupling could have such a strong impact on the pathology and symptoms of a brain disease as devastating as Alzheimer's. Researchers theorize that intense social interactions build "brain reserve," which increases resistance to memory loss and Alzheimer's. (See "Build 'Cognitive Reserve,'" page 77.) But for the moment, why singles are so at risk is still largely a mystery.

What to do? If you have a spouse or significant other, consider yourself lucky. If you don't, find one or compensate by forming strong social ties among a large circle of friends and relatives. All such socializing appears to keep brains happier and healthier and Alzheimer's at a more comfortable distance.

60

KNOW THE DANGERS OF **MEAT**

Too much meat primes your brain
for Alzheimer's

The more meat you eat, the more likely you are to have dementia," concluded a large British study of fifteen thousand older people in seven countries. Generally, meat eaters were about 20 percent more prone to dementia than those who never ate meat, said Emiliano Albanese, PhD, at King's College London, who conducted the study. Recent research at Columbia University in New York identified red meat and organ meat as culprits that raised the odds of Alzheimer's in a group of older people. Researchers at Loma Linda University in California reported that heavy meat eaters were more than twice as likely to develop dementia as vegetarians.

This should come as no surprise. Meat is guilty of inducing conditions incriminated in Alzheimer's. One example: inflammation. Meat is a major source of arachidonic acid, a known instigator of inflammation. Further, cooking meat typically produces very toxic chemicals called heterocyclic amines, or

HCAs. These are free radicals that viciously attack cells, causing oxidative damage, acknowledged as an underlying cause of age-related memory decline and Alzheimer's. Incidentally, HCAs also promote cancer. They form deep in the interior of the meat from a chemical reaction between heat and proteins in the animal flesh. Thus, HCAs cannot be scraped away. Further, meat is a major source of heme iron, and studies show that excess iron in the brain promotes neurodegeneration and dementia.

Then there are the dreaded nitrosamines, which can form in meat cured with sodium nitrite and in the body after eating such meats. These include ham, hot dogs, bacon, salami, bologna, pastrami, and all kinds of cold cuts. A recent study published in the *Journal of Alzheimer's Disease* tied the rising rates of deaths from Alzheimer's (as well as Parkinson's and diabetes) directly to increasing exposure to nitrosamines. "It was so shocking," says lead researcher Suzanne de la Monte, MD, a neuropathologist at Brown University's Warren Alpert Medical School in Providence. "You need to be really careful to avoid this stuff as much as possible." She suspected the hazard after studying a nitrosamine-like drug called streptozotocin, which can induce Alzheimer's in experimental animals. She wondered if nitrosamines from meat might do the same thing. She believes they do.

What to do? Limit the amount of red meat you eat; that means beef, pork, veal, and lamb, and particularly processed cured meats—ham, cold cuts, hot dogs, and bacon. All may set the stage for the progression of brain damage, leading to more rapid memory decline, dementia, and Alzheimer's. What about poultry? It is also considered meat, but it was identified by Columbia University researchers as a food that helped deter, not promote, Alzheimer's. Thus, it's okay to use poultry as a substitute for red meat, although fish is preferable.

61

CONSIDER **MEDICAL MARIJUANA**

Controversial, yes, but could it help prevent Alzheimer's?

An idea may seem wacky, absurd, or politically incorrect, but if there's legitimate science behind it, it may show up on the Alzheimer Research Forum's lively website (www .alzforum.org), which is dominated by heavy hitters in brain research. They thrive on unconventional postings that spark new thinking about Alzheimer's—like the case of the grandma with dementia who accidentally ate brownies containing marijuana. Instead of becoming worse, as feared, she became more lucid—each of the four times she ate them.

Whether the anecdote is true is unknown. But recent studies from leading institutions do show that chemicals in cannabis (marijuana's botanical name) can slow pathological brain changes in aging animals and even help them regain lost memory.

The Scripps Research Institute in California concluded that marijuana's active ingredient, THC (delta-9-tetrahydro-cannabinol), performs much like popular anti-Alzheimer's pharmaceuticals, but far better. In test-tube studies, THC blocked the formation of brain-clogging amyloid plaques 88 percent better than Aricept and 93 percent better than Cognex.

Giving old rats a synthetic THC-like chemical improved their memories, says Gary L. Wenk, PhD, a professor of psychology and neuroscience at Ohio State University. It helped rejuvenate certain brain functioning. Wenk credits marijuana's strong anti-inflammatory effects. Inflammation in the brain, he says, is a major villain in Alzheimer's, and THC penetrates the blood-brain barrier better than any agent he has studied.

Researchers, of course, don't recommend using illegal marijuana to try to prevent or treat Alzheimer's. Instead, Wenk is looking for legal ways to get a very tiny dose of the anti-Alzheimer's agent into the brain without causing a psychoactive high. One possibility, he says, is to develop a medical marijuana patch that delivers a very low, nonpsychoactive dose of THC through the skin. He hopes it might help save people at high risk of Alzheimer's before inflammation and symptoms become advanced.

What to do? Actually, not much but keep an open mind, says Wenk. The use of legal medical marijuana and synthetic THC is expanding. In the mysterious and devastating world of Alzheimer's disease, we may need to consider "offbeat ideas," adds another scientist. In the meantime, you should not depend on smoking marijuana as a way to help prevent memory loss or Alzheimer's. Smoking either ordinary tobacco or marijuana is potentially harmful.

62

PRACTICE **MEDITATION**

It's a quiet way to build a bigger, better brain

People who meditate regularly tend to retain more brain gray matter, show more sustained attention, and suffer less cognitive decline as they age, says Giuseppe Pagnoni, PhD, an assistant professor of psychiatry at Emory University. Using sophisticated brain scans to determine subjects' total volume of gray matter, he found that nonmeditators had the decline in gray matter expected with aging. But remarkably, practitioners of Zen meditation did not! Further, those who meditated also performed better on a computerized test of sustained attention.

UCLA researchers agree that meditation may help "build a bigger brain." MRI scans revealed that people who had meditated ten to ninety minutes every day for five to forty-six years had larger volumes of gray matter in certain regions of the brain related to memory and emotions than control subjects who did not meditate. The differences in brain anatomy may help explain why people who consistently meditate have more positive emotions, retain emotional stability, and engage better in mindful behavior (that is, are more focused), say researchers. How meditation could so powerfully alter brain structure is mysterious. Theories: it might somehow increase the number of neurons, stimulate growth of larger neurons, or create a particular "wiring" pattern.

Still, curbing brain shrinkage, a typical consequence of aging, is not the only way meditation may preserve our brains as we get older. Meditation also can lower blood pressure; reduce stress, depression, and inflammation; improve blood glucose and insulin levels; and increase blood flow to the brain—all related to memory loss, cognitive impairment, and Alzheimer's.

Surprisingly, there is much scientific support for various types of meditation in staving off cognitive problems. Andrew Newberg, MD, at the University of Pennsylvania School of Medicine, showed that a daily twelve-minute session of a type of yoga meditation known as Kirtan Kriya for eight weeks dramatically increased brain blood flow in people ages fifty-two to seventy-seven with mild cognitive impairment. Particularly interesting, meditation increased activity in the brain's frontal lobe, which is involved in retrieving memories and is specifically targeted by Alzheimer's. Better scores on a memory test also showed that meditation improved cognitive functioning. "For the first time we are seeing scientific evidence that meditation enables the brain to actually strengthen itself… and may even prevent neurodegenerative diseases such as Alzheimer's," said Newberg.

What to do? If you are unfamiliar with meditation, explore various types to see which appeals to you. Techniques vary, sometimes incorporating a specific posture or mantra (repetition of a word or phrase) intended to produce a focused and relaxed state of awareness. Look for meditation centers in your area. You can also get books, audiotapes, and DVDs showing how to meditate.

For a quick orientation and scientific information, check out the website of the National Center for Complementary and Alternative Medicine of the National Institutes of Health: http://nccam.nih.gov/health/meditation. It supports research on the benefits of meditation, including mindfulness meditation and Transcendental Meditation (TM).

Faithfully practicing meditation for even a few minutes a day could help preserve your mental acuity as you age and cut your odds of getting Alzheimer's.

63

FOLLOW THE **MEDITERRANEAN DIET**

Leafy greens, olive oil, and a little vino help keep Alzheimer's away

The Mediterranean diet, no matter where you live, can help save your brain from memory deterioration and dementia. Studies consistently find that what the Greeks and Italians traditionally eat is truly brain food. Following this diet—rich in green leafy vegetables, fish, fruits, nuts, legumes, and a little vino—can cut your chances of Alzheimer's in half.

And the closer you follow the diet, the more dramatic the benefits to your aging brain. In a recent study by leading Alzheimer's researcher Nikolaos Scarmeas, MD, at Columbia University College of Physicians and Surgeons, the odds that older individuals with normal memory would develop mild cognitive impairment dropped by 28 percent in those who stuck closest to the Mediterranean diet, compared to those who strayed furthest from the diet. Even those who paid middling attention to the diet cut their risk of cognitive impairment by 17 percent.

The news is even better for people who fear that their mild memory loss might progress to Alzheimer's. Adhering most faithfully to the Mediterranean diet cut the odds of slipping into Alzheimer's by 48 percent—nearly in half!

What makes the Mediterranean diet so powerful is that it does not depend on just one food or a few nutrients. It is a rich menu of many complex brain benefactors. Scarmeas credits an array of antioxidants (including vitamins C and E and carotenoids) in olive oil, red wine, and fruits and vegetables, particularly tomatoes, onions, and garlic, with shielding brain cells from oxidative damage.

Many of the same foods fight inflammation, a culprit in Alzheimer's. A blood test for C-reactive protein (CRP), a measure of inflammation, showed that women who strictly followed the Mediterranean diet had 24 percent lower scores than those on an ordinary diet, according to Harvard doctors. Omega-3s in fatty fish are also strong anti-inflammatories. And olive oil, a staple of the Mediterranean diet, contains chemicals found to discourage the development of neurofibrillary tau tangles, a hallmark of Alzheimer's.

What to do? Go Mediterranean with a passion. Here's Scarmeas's description of such a diet: "The traditional Mediterranean diet is characterized by high consumption of plant foods (vegetables, fruits, legumes, and cereals); high intake of olive oil as the principal source of monounsaturated fat, but low intake of saturated fat; moderate intake of fish; low to moderate intake of dairy products; low consumption of meat and poultry; and wine consumed in low to moderate amounts, normally with meals." The Mediterranean diet, he adds, includes sweets and red meat only two to three times a month.

64

RECOGNIZE **MEMORY PROBLEMS**

Is it normal aging or Alzheimer's?

By middle age, virtually everybody's memory has slipped, requiring more time to learn, process, and retrieve information. It's normal. So the big question is, how can you tell if your memory is declining normally or accelerating toward a rendezvous with Alzheimer's?

Fascinating new research by Barry Reisberg, MD, director of the Fisher Alzheimer's Disease Program at New York University's Langone Medical Center, finds that you may be your own best diagnostician. Here's why: Long before the onset of dementia, he explains, you are likely to pass through two memory-loss stages. One is called mild cognitive impairment (MCI), or "early Alzheimer's," and typically precedes dementia by seven years or so. About 10 to 15 percent of people with mild cognitive problems go on to a diagnosis of Alzheimer's every year. Many do not; some even improve, and there is no simple, reliable test for MCI. Clues are: getting lost when traveling to unfamiliar places, being unable to come up with words and names, and having trouble recalling a passage just read in a book. People at this stage commonly have confirmable brain pathology.

The other, more recently recognized memory-loss stage, called "subjective cognitive impairment" (SCI), shows up about fifteen years before MCI surfaces. The sole symptom of SCI: you sense that your memory is in trouble, but objective tests don't show it. You can't remember names or where you put your car keys as well as you used to. This earliest SCI stage of memory loss, "when the patient knows, but the doctor doesn't," foreshadows dementia by more than twenty years, says Reisberg.

Only you can spot SCI. If you are sixty or older, are you concerned about your memory? Do you think your memory is much less sharp than it was a year ago? If so, it's possible that your memory is declining abnormally, and you may have SCI. Before you panic, you need to know that SCI is also associated with treatable disorders such as depression, anxiety, thyroid dysfunction, vitamin B_{12} deficiency, aneurysm, head injury, and medications. So SCI is far from a sure path to dementia and may be reversible.

However, Reisberg says your own suspicion that your memory is failing is right about half the time. He tracked 213 cognitively normal adults in their sixties for seven years; some worried they were losing their memory, others did not. Among the worriers, 54 percent went on to experience MCI or dementia compared with only 15 percent who had no self-confessed memory worries. Even so, 46 percent of those with SCI did not develop symptomatic memory loss during the study, showing that your own foreboding of memory failure does not always mean you are speeding toward dementia.

What to do? If you recognize memory decline, think of it as an opportunity to intervene and arrest progression. The earlier you are on the case, the better, and you have a long time (a decade or two) in which to take action. First, have a thorough medical checkup to find out if your memory problems could be due to a treatable medical condition. (See "Get the Right Diagnosis," page 95.) If not, consult a neurologist, preferably one who specializes in geriatrics or dementia.

It is essential not to discount the earliest memory complaints in yourself or others. Once memory loss progresses to MCI, the affected person begins to deny that anything is wrong. The earlier memory decline is recognized, the sooner you may be able to interrupt it and rescue a brain from dementia.

65

KEEP **MENTALLY ACTIVE**

"Use it or lose it" is a mantra against Alzheimer's

What if you could cut your odds of ever developing dementia in half or even by two thirds—just by keeping your brain stimulated in your spare time? You can, according to research at Albert Einstein College of Medicine at Yeshiva University.

No matter how much you used your brain in the past or how much cognitive reserve you have on tap to deter Alzheimer's, staying mentally active as you age is one of the most powerful things you can do to keep dementia at a distance, says Charles B. Hall, PhD, a professor at Einstein. The more brain-stimulating activities you do every day, he says, "the longer the delay in memory decline."

Hall studied the leisure activities of five hundred elderly men and women in the so-called Bronx Aging Study. All were free of dementia at ages seventy-five to eighty-five when the study began in 1983. Over time, about 20 percent developed dementia. The striking fact: those who engaged in the most mentally stimulating activities—such as reading, writing, doing crossword puzzles, playing board or card games, participating in group discussions, or playing music—were the least apt to "experience the rapid memory loss associated with dementia." Doing only one brain activity every day delayed the onset of memory loss and dementia by two months! Hall's conclusion: "We found that the more brain-stimulating activities you do and the more often you do them, the better off you are."

That is true worldwide. Australian neuroscientist Michael Valenzuela, PhD, and colleagues at Prince of Wales Hospital in Sydney analyzed twenty-two studies involving twenty-nine thousand people and concluded that high mental activity levels reduced the risk of dementia by 46 percent compared to low activity levels. The benefits of increased mental activity were particularly outstanding in late life.

Researchers can measure the impact of mental activity on the brain. Using MRIs and PET scans, scientists can directly link mental activity to increases in gray matter and neurotropic factors—small proteins that nourish nerve cells, including BDNF (brain-derived neurotropic factor), which some researchers jokingly call Miracle-Gro for nerve cells. Mental activity encourages the birth and survival of new brain cells and synapses (transmission centers) and possibly even blood vessels. In short, mental activity improves both the anatomy and the functioning of the brain.

And there's a risk if you let up on mental activity. Scientists have discovered that cutting down on mental stimulation causes certain aspects of both cognitive functioning and brain structures to stall or go into reverse, proving that if you don't use it, you do lose it. Thus, mental inactivity can bring you closer to memory impairment and dementia.

What to do? Keep your brain active for a lifetime, particularly as you grow older. That means engaging in all kinds of leisure activities that stimulate your brain. Remember, the more mental activity, the more your brain thrives and grows. If you do one or two mental activities a day, up it to three or four or more. (See also "Build 'Cognitive Reserve,'" page 77, "Do Something New," page 203, and "Surround Yourself with Stimulation," page 245.)

66

TAKE **MULTIVITAMINS**

They can slow aging and delay Alzheimer's

If you stayed forever young, Alzheimer's would probably not be a problem. The driving force behind the disease is increasing age. So, what if you could slow the aging process and thus delay the likelihood of cognitive decline and Alzheimer's?

Exciting research from the National Institute of Environmental Health Sciences suggests that may be possible simply by taking multivitamins and antioxidants. Their findings are based on measuring the length of protective caps on the tips of chromosomes, called telomeres, described by one scientist as "like the plastic tips on the ends of shoelaces." The length of these telomeres indicates how fast a person is aging biologically. Shorter telomeres predict accelerated aging, earlier death, and a higher risk of age-related chronic diseases, including Alzheimer's.

Researchers at Harvard Medical School found a striking connection between telomere length and Alzheimer's. Women with shorter telomeres in blood leukocytes were twelve times more likely to have mild cognitive impairment, a prelude to Alzheimer's, than women with longer telomeres. MRIs also showed more brain shrinkage in women with shorter telomeres.

The big question: what lengthens or shortens telomeres? Typically, agents that cause inflammation and free-radical damage to cells shorten telomeres. These villains include air pollution, cigarette smoking, obesity, high homocysteine, and a sedentary lifestyle—all risk factors for Alzheimer's. The good news: micronutrients, including antioxidants such as vitamins C and E, as well as vitamin D and folic acid, tend to counteract telomere shortening.

That's why investigators at the National Institute of Environmental Health Sciences decided to find out if people who took multivitamins and antioxidants had longer, younger-looking telomeres. The resounding answer: yes! Women who regularly took multivitamins had 5 percent longer telomeres than non–supplement takers. The price women paid for not taking multivitamins was shortened telomeres that looked about ten years older.

Compared with non–supplement takers, women who took a "once-a-day Centrum-type multivitamin" for at least five years had 3 percent longer telomeres. Telomeres were *8 percent* longer in women who habitually took a multivitamin-antioxidant combination with high doses of extra antioxidants, such as vitamin C and vitamin E.

Further, women who took an individual B_{12} tablet daily had 6 percent longer telomeres. But women who took a stand-alone iron pill had *9 percent shorter* telomeres. Excess iron produces free-radical damage to cells, which may account for this alarming finding.

Several studies show that combinations of a variety of vitamins and minerals are more likely than single nutrients to optimally protect an aging brain. Example: a potent blend of thirty-four antioxidants, taken for four months, improved memory performance in a large group of seniors (aged fifty to seventy-five) without dementia. The blend included alpha lipoic acid, vitamin C, beta carotene, folic acid, magnesium, nicotinamide, vitamins B$_6$ and B$_{12}$, and mixed forms of vitamin E. The controlled double blind study was conducted by researchers at a private institute in New Mexico and the University of Pittsburgh.

What to do? Start taking a daily multivitamin if you don't already. A once-a-day low-dose multi that contains no iron should help slow aging in your brain. But for much greater antiaging brain protection, choose a super-multivitamin formula high in antioxidants, notably vitamins C and E, as well as a variety of other nutrients. You can find high-antioxidant formulations of multivitamins on the Internet and in retail stores.

Important: Don't take iron supplements if you are an adult man or a postmenopausal woman unless recommended by a medical professional for a specific reason. Beware of supplements that contain copper if you eat a high-fat diet. (See "Keep Copper and Iron Out of Your Brain," page 82. Also see "Take Folic Acid," page 127, and "Don't Neglect Vitamin D," page 273.)

67

BUILD STRONG **MUSCLES**

Weak muscles may signal Alzheimer's ahead

It's not enough to concentrate entirely on aerobic exercise to keep your brain in shape. Building strong muscles also helps keep your brain Alzheimer's-free. Some of the same pathology underlies both weakening muscles and diminishing cognitive function, experts believe, and building up muscles translates into improved brain functioning.

In research at Rush University Medical Center in Chicago, Patricia Boyle, PhD, discovered that older people with weaker muscles were more vulnerable targets of cognitive decline and Alzheimer's. Those with the strongest muscles overall were 61 percent less likely to face a diagnosis of Alzheimer's, compared with those with the weakest muscles.

Which muscular areas were most apt to predict Alzheimer's? A weaker hand grip and weaker chest and abdominal muscles that control breathing, says Boyle. She previously noted that a decline in grip strength of one pound per year over five years raised Alzheimer's risk 9 percent.

Also, as older people become increasingly frail, their risk of Alzheimer's rises. Signs of frailty are loss of muscle mass (sarcopenia), decreased grip strength, less physical activity, exhaustion, and weight loss—a drop of over ten pounds or 5 percent of weight in the past year.

Fortunately, strength training can help counter muscle loss and improve cognition in older people. Women ages sixty-five to seventy-five who worked out with dumbbells and weight machines an hour or two a week for a year scored higher on tests of specific cognitive functions, according to a study by Teresa Liu-Ambrose, PhD, at the University of British Columbia in Vancouver. These women improved by 10 to 12 percent in so-called executive function—the ability to plan and execute tasks, make decisions, resolve conflicts, and focus—in comparison to similar women who did less demanding toning and balance exercises.

Similarly, sedentary men over age sixty-five who did six months of resistance exercise on specific equipment (chest press, leg press, vertical traction, abdominal crunch, leg curl, and lower back) improved on tests of cognition whether the intensity of the exercise was moderate or high.

What to do? No doubt about it: you should build up your muscles and keep them strong. Walk thirty minutes a day to build up leg muscles. Engage in moderate weight lifting and other resistance-type exercises to increase the size and strength of specific muscles. Experts recommend eight to ten strength-training exercises (eight to fifteen repetitions each) two or three times a week. You may want to work out with weights and on machines at a gym. But you can also build stronger muscles by doing simple exercises at home. An hour a couple of times a week at the gym or daily sessions of ten to twenty minutes at home can make a big difference.

You can find excellent video examples of types of exercise, including "Strength Training at Home," at www.youtube.com; enter the search term "Exercise is Medicine," which is a video series created by the American College of Sports Medicine. The videos are also at www.acsm.org.

68

TAKE A **NATURE HIKE**

It can calm your mind and improve
short-term memory

You can spend an hour either walking down an urban street, with all its distractions, or strolling around a botanical garden, taking in nature. Marc Berman, a neuroscientist at the University of Michigan, tested the effects of walking each route on short-term memory and ability to focus. Based on previous evidence, he expected a nature walk to be a better brain booster. It was. In fact, he concluded that "interacting with nature had similar effects on the brain to meditating."

Specifically, Berman sent thirty-eight people on two one-hour walks: one along the busy main streets of Ann Arbor and the other around the University of Michigan's Matthaei Botanical Gardens and Nichols Arboretum. He gave the subjects memory tests before and after the walks. It turned out that walking in the serene surroundings of trees and plants restored attention and even improved short-term memory by a remarkable

20 percent. Memory scores did not change after the city walk. Clearly, it was a victory for nature over urban clamor.

Further, the benefits were the same whether people walked in eighty-degree summer heat or twenty-five-degree January cold. People "didn't have to enjoy the walk to get the benefits," Berman points out.

He explains his findings with this psychological theory: urban stimuli fatigue the brain's attention faculties; they are restored when the brain can relax in a natural setting. Berman also found that just viewing pictures of scenery for ten minutes improved memory and attention.

What to do? It certainly makes sense to take walks on nature trails and in parks and gardens. You get not only the physical activity that protects your brain but an added bonus of meditation-like relaxation and a boost of short-term memory—the type most vulnerable to Alzheimer's damage. Although Berman tested younger people, he thinks nature walks would have an even more profound memory benefit for older people who already have some impairment.

69

DO SOMETHING **NEW**

Your brain lights up when you have a new thought or experience

Learn a new word, and the hippocampus in your brain glows before it passes on the information for permanent transcription. Your brain is activated by novelty, says Arnold Scheibel, MD, former director of the Brain Research Institute at UCLA. The brain is hardwired to become alert to anything new and exotic, he explains. "It's an evolutionary survival mechanism that developed when we had to look out for predators."

The "novelty response," as psychologists call it, can help your brain survive the threat of Alzheimer's. Having a new thought or experience stimulates dendritic growth in nerve cells, expanding brain volume. And brains of lab animals set free to explore an open field for the first time squirt out extra acetylcholine, the so-called memory chemical. That's why people should not only remain mentally active, but also "take up *new* pursuits," says Scheibel. Seeking the new actually builds brain structure and function.

Any mental activity intended to help prevent Alzheimer's must be stimulating, which usually means new, agrees Robert S. Wilson, PhD, a neuropsychologist at Rush University Medical Center in Chicago. Breezing through one more crossword puzzle with your mind on autopilot does not wake up lazy brain cells, he says. Going on to learn something new does.

In a series of studies, brain researchers at Case Western Reserve University in Cleveland identified which leisure-time mental activities are most likely to fend off Alzheimer's. Number one: "novelty-seeking" activities, followed by "exchange of ideas" activities. Moreover, people who were less intellectually and physically active in their twenties through fifties were 250 percent more likely to have Alzheimer's in late life.

And guess which leisure activity was most apt to turn your brain toward Alzheimer's? Watching television. The startling fact: for every hour a day that people watched TV in midlife (ages forty to fifty-nine), their risk of Alzheimer's jumped by 30 percent. Lead researcher Robert Friedland, MD, agrees that television can be intellectually stimulating, but not if people watch it in a semiconscious state. Further, passive TV watching replaces mentally stimulating leisure activities.

What to do? Anything new. The possibilities are endless: Learn a new word every day. Take up quilting, piano playing, tap dancing, painting, jigsaw puzzles, sightseeing. Visit museums. Learn a new language, a new card game, or a board game. Join a book club. Go to adult education classes. Learn Photoshop on the computer. Do anything you have not done before. And when you are proficient, go on to something else new. Seek out novelty your entire life.

Many researchers believe that years of activating brain cells by embracing novelty and learning helps create a strong defense against intellectual decline and Alzheimer's. Challenge your mind all day long.

70

GET ENOUGH **NIACIN**

This common vitamin may rescue you from Alzheimer's

A modest little B vitamin called niacin (vitamin B_3) is making big waves in Alzheimer's research. Here's what happened after University of California, Irvine, investigators put an over-the-counter form of niacin called nicotinamide in the drinking water of mice genetically destined to get Alzheimer's: they didn't. Their memories—short-term and long-term—performed normally. They zipped through water mazes and other cognitive tests just as well as mice without the Alzheimer's genes. Nicotinamide even boosted memory in normal mice. Those not sucking up niacin did develop Alzheimer's-like memory loss.

When researchers examined the brains of the nicotinamide-fed mice, they saw why there had been no memory failure. The niacin had flushed out some of the toxic stuff in neurons that makes the incapacitating tau tangles seen in Alzheimer's.

The vitamin also bucked up the cellular scaffolding, or "highways," that carry information, enabling neurons to stay alive and prevent symptoms.

Tests using 1,500 mg of nicotinamide twice daily in Alzheimer's patients are under way, says study coauthor Frank LaFerla, PhD, a professor of neurobiology and the director of the university's Institute for Memory Impairments and Neurological Disorders.

More good niacin news: Martha Clare Morris, ScD, at the Rush Institute for Healthy Aging in Chicago, says that eating niacin-packed foods may fend off Alzheimer's, too — the more niacin, the less cognitive decline after age sixty-five. In Morris's study, people eating the most niacin, an average of 22.4 mg daily, compared with the least, 12.6 mg, cut their odds of developing Alzheimer's by 80 percent.

What to do? It makes total sense to eat niacin-rich foods, such as canned or fresh tuna, chicken and turkey breast, salmon, swordfish, halibut, sardines, peanuts, and cereals such as Cheerios, All-Bran, and Total. Check food labels. It's not hard to get a brain-saving quota of more than 22 mg of niacin a day. Multivitamins typically contain niacin; for example, a daily dose of Centrum Silver provides 14 mg of niacin.

As for taking nonprescription nicotinamide to prevent Alzheimer's? It's too early to recommend it, says LaFerla. He points out that the best preventive dose is unknown but is bound to be high, possibly causing side effects such as headaches, dizziness, liver damage, and increased blood sugar. If you take high doses for any reason, you should be monitored by a medical professional, he cautions. Even though the upper safe dose is 3,000 mg a day, some people do not tolerate it well and could get in trouble.

71

THINK ABOUT A **NICOTINE PATCH**

It might keep your memory loss from progressing to Alzheimer's

Sometime in late middle age, some people begin to slip into a condition often referred to as "mild cognitive impairment" (MCI). It means your memory is becoming worse and your brain is showing signs of damage that may progress to Alzheimer's pathology. MCI is a transitional period between normal cognition and Alzheimer's dementia that could last ten years or so. Scientists are seeking new interventions that will stop these mild cognitive problems from progressing to dementia, which happens in 10 to 15 percent of MCI cases a year.

That's why Paul A. Newhouse, MD, the associate director for research at the University of Vermont Center on Aging, asked seventy-four nonsmokers age fifty-five and older who had mild MCI to wear a nicotine patch for a year. You may be surprised to learn that nicotine can boost the functioning of acetylcholine, a neurotransmitter typically diminished in the brains of people with MCI and Alzheimer's. Thus, it may improve learning, memory, and focus. In animal studies, nicotine also reduced brain levels of toxic beta-amyloid and blocked its ability to impair cognition.

Newhouse knew that nicotine looked like a good bet to help thwart cognitive decline. The problem, of course: when nicotine is inhaled in cigarette smoke, it is addictive, and smoking can lead to cancer, vascular dementia, and other diseases. So why not deliver the potential memory booster through a nonaddictive skin patch that doles out small, regular doses of nicotine? It worked.

In Newhouse's double-blind study, those with impaired memory who wore the nicotine patch improved on cognitive measures, including delayed-word-recall accuracy, speed of memory, and reaction time. The cognitive boost was greater in carriers of two copies of the ApoE4 gene, a prime risk factor for Alzheimer's.

There were no downsides to the nicotine patch, says Newhouse, and on the upside, it lowered blood pressure. He is enthusiastic about the prospect that wearing a nicotine patch may be "one way to treat the earliest signs of memory loss."

What to do? First, what not to do: do not smoke cigarettes to get nicotine into your brain. Not only is the smoke hazardous, but the sporadic hits of nicotine you get from smoking are not long lasting. But if you are in the early stages of age-related memory loss, you might want to think about a nicotine patch to see if it helps. The dose in each transdermal nicotine patch used in Newhouse's study was the same as that in patches used by people to try to quit smoking. This small dose of nicotine was also free of major side effects and did not contribute to dependency. Talk it over with your doctor if you are interested.

72

BE CAUTIOUS ABOUT **NSAIDs**

Nobody knows whether they help prevent Alzheimer's

Investigators are hedging their bets on recommending NSAIDs (nonsteroidal anti-inflammatory drugs) to prevent Alzheimer's. Theoretically, the drugs are appealing, since suppressing inflammation, which they do, should limit Alzheimer's damage. And their promise has generated excitement among researchers. But in reality, nobody really knows if they work.

In a first big test, NSAIDs failed miserably. The Alzheimer's Disease Anti-Inflammatory Prevention Trial (ADAPT), a controlled trial involving twenty-five hundred Americans over age seventy at high risk for Alzheimer's, found no evidence that two NSAIDs—celecoxib (Celebrex) and naproxen (Aleve)—prevented Alzheimer's after two years of use. The study was suspended. However, follow-up data suggest that protection did kick in a few years later. An analysis published in October 2009 claims that taking naproxen actually reduced new cases of Alzheimer's by an amazing two thirds. This means that a two-year use of the anti-inflammatory had a delayed preventive impact on older brains several years later. Experts unrelated to the study say that if this is true, it's excellent news, but for the moment the jury is out. The study goes on.

Then there's ibuprofen, also sold as Advil and Motrin, which looks good in several studies. Boston University researchers who analyzed Department of Veterans Affairs medical records of just under two hundred fifty thousand patients concluded that regularly taking ibuprofen for more than four years cut the risk of developing Alzheimer's by 44 percent. Taking any NSAID, including ibuprofen, for more than four years reduced Alzheimer's odds by about one fourth. Taking NSAIDs for one to four years cut the odds 10 percent, while taking them for less than one year had no effect.

Researchers believe ibuprofen may be superior to other NSAIDs in preventing Alzheimer's because it is not just an anti-inflammatory. Studies show it also reduces beta-amyloid, that sticky stuff in brain cells said to incite Alzheimer's.

And what about low-dose aspirin? It may help, according to a Dutch study, but because of its anticoagulant properties, not its anti-inflammatory ones. Then again, it may not, say British researchers who found no anti-Alzheimer's benefits from low-dose aspirin taken for five years by people over age fifty.

On the other hand, a recent University of Washington study suggests that various NSAIDs may *raise* the Alzheimer's risk about 30 percent. "It's hard to explain," says one researcher, who thinks NSAIDs will turn out to help prevent Alzheimer's in some people, especially those with the high-risk ApoE4 gene. "But we don't know yet," he adds.

What to do? If you are taking aspirin for cardiovascular reasons, continue under your doctor's direction and hope it also helps stave off strokes and dementia. Experts do not recommend taking NSAIDs, including aspirin and ibuprofen, specifically to ward off Alzheimer's. The evidence is still uncertain, and the risks, particularly of intestinal bleeding, could outweigh the benefits.

73

GO NUTS OVER **NUTS**

A daily handful of almonds or walnuts may fend off Alzheimer's

Nuts have some of the same antioxidant powers as fruits and vegetables in protecting the brain from memory loss and Alzheimer's. James Joseph, PhD, at Tufts University, who discovered that blueberries reversed memory loss in aging rats, has called walnuts "blueberries in a shell." Rats fed walnuts also became "younger and smarter," he said. In people, an ounce a day (seven to nine walnuts) may help delay the onset of Alzheimer's and other dementias, he declared.

Walnuts curb oxidative damage to brain cells, a known cause of neuronal death leading to Alzheimer's; fight inflammation; and even stimulate the birth of new neurons and increase the communication powers of old ones. Walnuts, like blueberries, rejuvenate the very structure of brain cells, enabling old rats to perform feats of memory and learning just as well as younger ones.

Moreover, test-tube research at Baldwin-Wallace College

in Berea, Ohio, showed that a walnut extract blocked the aggregation of toxic beta-amyloid, a first step toward Alzheimer's, and even broke up preformed clumps of the toxin already engaged in the process of killing brain cells.

Almonds are also a good bet to help save you from Alzheimer's. When fed the human equivalent of a handful of almonds a day, mice with Alzheimer's-type plaques did better on memory and learning tests than mice fed only their usual chow, according to research by Neelima Chauhan, PhD, at the University of Illinois, Chicago.

Further, the amount of toxic beta-amyloid in the brains of the almond-eating rodents actually shrank. Chauhan explains that almonds have activity similar to that of Alzheimer's drugs called cholinesterase inhibitors (for example, Aricept), which increase levels of the neurotransmitter acetylcholine. That doesn't mean eating almonds can treat or cure Alzheimer's by any means, but it might help prevent the progression of the disease, says Chauhan.

Since most nuts have similar nutrients and antioxidants, it's likely that many varieties have anti-Alzheimer's activity but have not yet been tested. It's well known that nuts in general, and almonds and walnuts in particular, are good for the heart and cardiovascular system. Walnuts, for example, help lower cholesterol and blood sugar, improve blood flow, and help fend off diabetes, says recent Yale University research.

What to do? Eat a handful of almonds or walnuts every day. No need to eat more, researchers say, or to be afraid that fatty nuts will make you gain weight. Actually, studies show that nuts tend to fill you up and help curb your appetite.

It's better to choose almonds with the skins on; the skin contains most of the nut's antioxidants. And don't hesitate to eat other kinds of nuts. Most are extremely high in antioxidants. Pecans actually rank first in antioxidants, followed by walnuts, hazelnuts, pistachios, almonds, peanuts (technically a legume), cashews, macadamia nuts, and Brazil nuts.

74

WORRY ABOUT MIDDLE-AGE **OBESITY**

Excess weight shrinks your brain and sets the stage for dementia

Unfortunately, your brain cares if you are fat. Researchers at UCLA and the University of Pittsburgh have the pictures to prove it. They did brain imaging of people in their seventies who were not cognitively impaired. Nevertheless, overweight and obese individuals had "severe brain degeneration" due to brain shrinkage, says Paul Thompson, PhD, a professor of neurology at UCLA. A shrunken brain is more vulnerable to cognitive decline.

Specifically, obese people had 8 percent less brain tissue and overweight people had 4 percent less brain tissue than normal-weight people. "That's a big loss of tissue," says Thompson, "putting you at much greater risk of Alzheimer's and other diseases that attack the brain." (Obese is defined as having a BMI—body mass index—of more than 30; overweight, a BMI between 25 and 30; and normal weight, a BMI between 18.5 and 25.)

Moreover, brain shrinkage occurred in areas of the brain that are targeted by Alzheimer's—in the frontal and temporal lobes, critical for planning and memory; the anterior cingulate gyrus, attention and executive functions; the hippocampus, long-term memory; and the basal ganglia, control of movement.

Here's how Thompson summed it up: "The brains of obese people looked sixteen years older and the brains of overweight people eight years older than those of normal-weight individuals."

It's not entirely clear how gaining pounds erases brain matter, but it's apt to happen over many years. That supports other evidence that being overweight and obese in midlife sets the stage for late-life dementia. Leading authority Rachel A. Whitmer, PhD, at Kaiser Permanente's Division of Research in Oakland, California, has shown that if you are obese at ages forty to forty-five, you are three times more likely to have Alzheimer's and five times more likely to have vascular dementia in your seventies and eighties than someone who was of normal weight during middle age. The best time to lose excess weight, especially belly fat, to prevent later cognitive loss is during midlife, she says.

What to do? When you see your weight creeping up, tackle the problem early, when you are young or middle-aged. That's when it probably makes the most difference. Oddly, being obese in old age (after seventy or seventy-five) does not raise the risk of Alzheimer's, something researchers dub "the obesity paradox." Nevertheless, don't neglect exercise if you are overweight later in life. Exercise is magical at stimulating better cognitive functioning and possibly delays the onset of Alzheimer's at any age, especially if you are obese or overweight. (Also see "Watch Your Waist," page 276.)

75

GET HELP FOR **OBSTRUCTIVE SLEEP APNEA**

It can cause brain damage and memory loss

About twenty million Americans have a sleep disorder in which they gasp for air, emitting loud bursts of snoring, sometimes hundreds of times a night. It happens when muscles in your throat and mouth relax, allowing your tongue to slide back toward your throat, blocking your windpipe and cutting off oxygen. This is called "obstructive sleep apnea," and most people consider it a mild inconvenience and worry little about it.

But it can have serious consequences for your brain, researchers at UCLA have discovered. Using MRI brain scans, they detected a loss of brain tissue in sleep apnea patients similar to that seen in Alzheimer's brains. In fact, a specific area of the brain involved in memory was 20 percent smaller than normal in sleep apnea sufferers. This is "a sizable cell loss" showing that patients have suffered long-lasting "serious brain injury that disrupts memory and thinking," concluded principal investigator Ronald Harper, PhD, a professor of neurobiology at UCLA's David Geffen School of Medicine.

Harper theorizes that lack of oxygen is to blame for neuronal loss. He explains that during an apnea episode, brain blood vessels constrict, starving nerve cells of oxygen and causing them to die. At the same time, the process triggers inflammation, further damaging brain tissue.

Researchers are not saying that sleep apnea causes Alzheimer's, but rather that it appears to worsen cognitive decline. About 70 to 80 percent of Alzheimer's patients have sleep apnea, say researchers at the University of California, San Diego. In fact, a team led by Sonia Ancoli-Israel, PhD, a professor of psychiatry, found that treating sleep apnea in Alzheimer's patients using "continuous positive airway pressure," or CPAP, improved their cognitive test scores.

What to do? If you believe you have sleep apnea, have it medically diagnosed, preferably at a sleep clinic, and get treatment. UCLA's Harper says the earlier the diagnosis and treatment, the better for stalling brain damage and potential memory loss. Normal sleep apnea patients without dementia have also had cognitive boosts from CPAP treatment, which involves wearing a breathing device over the mouth and/or nose to provide a constant supply of pressurized air during sleep.

76

GO FOR **OLIVE OIL**

Its secret ingredient blocks the genesis of Alzheimer's

talians, of course, are always giddy over olive oil. It is the secret to almost everything good—a strong heart, dense bones, lower blood pressure, better blood cholesterol and coagulation, and a stronger brain more resistant to cognitive decline and Alzheimer's as you grow old. Countless Italians will testify to it, and studies verify it.

One example: among a group of 278 elderly southern Italians, the odds of age-related memory decline and cognitive functioning dropped fully one third in those who ate the most olive oil. They downed a daily average of three tablespoons of presumably extra-virgin olive oil. It worked, say researchers, because olive oil helps maintain the "structural integrity of neuronal membranes" and contains antioxidants that deflect free-radical hits destined to cripple and kill brain cells.

But science has now discovered another mighty weapon in extra-virgin olive oil—a compound called oleocanthal, which zaps the genesis of Alzheimer's from day one. According to researchers at Northwestern University's Cognitive Neurology and Alzheimer's Disease Center and the Monell Chemical Senses Center in Philadelphia, oleocanthal helps prevent toxic baby blobs of beta-amyloid, known as oligomers, from attaching to nerve cell synapses and setting off destructive forces that lead to cell death and eventual Alzheimer's. Even small amounts of oleocanthal appear to counteract this Alzheimer's process in test-tube studies. Further, the olive oil compound has anti-inflammatory powers that help counteract Alzheimer's damage.

Among a large group of elderly French men and women who also embrace the Mediterranean diet, those who ate the most olive oil had a lower risk of cognitive problems. Compared with non–olive oil users, those who used olive oil for both dressings and cooking were 17 percent less likely to expe rience a decline in visual memory and verbal fluency over a four-year period.

What to do? Make extra-virgin olive oil numero uno in your kitchen. Olive oil, which is highly monounsaturated, is part of what makes the Mediterranean diet so friendly to aging brains. There is no set quota of olive oil you need to consume. Just substitute it for other salad and cooking oils, particularly pro-inflammatory corn and soyabean oils. Other occasionally okay oils include canola, almond, walnut, avocado, and macadamia nut. Still, using *only* olive oil, preferably less-processed extra-virgin oil, means you never even have to think about it, so you can never go wrong.

77

BEWARE OF **OMEGA-6 FAT**

It's a vicious source of inflammation and brain cell death

One of the best ways to ruin your brain—and your heart and entire cardiovascular system—is to pig out on a type of fatty acid called omega-6, most often found in corn oil, soybean oil, salad dressings, and margarine.

Unfortunately, the Western diet is overflowing with omega-6 fats. We eat at least five times more than we should for optimal brain functioning. Most omega-6s show up in highly processed and fast foods, contributing to their reputation as junk food. Essentially, omega-6 fats stimulate processes that pile up destructive Alzheimer's gunk, such as beta-amyloid proteins, in brain cells.

The greatest sin of omega-6 fatty acids: they throw off incendiary agents called prostaglandins and arachidonic acid, which spread inflammation throughout the brain, resulting in a massacre of neurons. Some scientists consider these inflammatory agents neurotoxins.

Much evidence indicts omega-6s in brain degeneration. A large Dutch study found that older men who ate the most omega-6 fat, primarily in margarine, baking fats, and sauces, were 75 percent more likely to be cognitively impaired than men who ate the least. Among eight thousand French men and women, regular consumers of omega-6-rich oils were twice as apt to develop dementia, notably when they did not offset the overload of omega-6 with the omega-3 fat in fish.

It's important to know that eating lots of omega-6 fat can undo the brain protection provided by omega-3-rich fish. Animal studies consistently show that even if you feed your brain loads of fish oil, you reduce its protection against memory decline and dementia if you also pour on lots of omega-6s. Only by cutting back on omega-6 fat, with its ability to set your brain on fire, can you optimally stave off neuronal destruction and dementia.

What to do? Stop brain inflammation now by cutting down on omega-6-packed corn oil, soybean oil, and regular safflower and sunflower seed oils (high oleic, as noted on the label, is okay). Since omega-6s per se are not specifically listed on labels, your best precaution is to use primarily extra-virgin olive oil.

Also load up on omega-3 to offset the bad omega-6. Based on current consumption of omega-6 and omega-3 fat, one expert says that one half tablespoon of soybean or corn oil contains the maximum amount of hazardous omega-6 fat you should consume in a day.

78

KNOW YOUR **PLAQUES AND TANGLES**

Amyloid and tau are the twins of destruction

To confirm Alzheimer's, specialists look for two telltale signs in the brain: "plaques" of a small protein called beta-amyloid and "neurofibrillary tangles" of a protein called tau. These accumulate because brain cells produce too much and flush away too little. Over time, the two toxins mangle brain structure, muck up transmissions, cause neurons to die, and leave brain matter to shrink. Communications cease, memory goes cold, and dementia appears. These plaques and tangles, which can now be detected in living brains by sophisticated PET scans, begin building up a decade or more before the symptoms of Alzheimer's appear. Together beta-amyloid and tau are the unique signature of Alzheimer's.

So goes the major prevailing theory of the underlying cause of Alzheimer's. Most research focuses on defining and defeating these two devils in an effort to stop the earliest stages of disease that can lead to dementia. Although some researchers dispute their dominant importance, beta-amyloid and tau currently hold center stage as the twins of destruction and the targets for preventing Alzheimer's.

How does beta-amyloid do its damage? It is released when synapses (infinitesimal gaps between neurons) fire to transmit messages between nerve cells. Everybody's brain cells rapidly produce and eliminate beta-amyloid every day, and its levels fluctuate constantly—that's normal. Trouble comes when, for genetic and other reasons, the brain accumulates too much. Excessive beta-amyloid forms dangerous floating clumps called oligomers, which can morph into abnormal plaques, leaving a trail of silent synapses and dying neurons. Recent findings suggest that the oligomers, rather than the plaques, are the prime villains in the disease.

Tau tangles are a more recently discovered sidekick villain in Alzheimer's and other types of dementia. When normal, tau smooths the way for the transmission of signals along axons and dendrites—stringy protrusions that connect the networks of billions of neurons to one another. In some brains, aging changes cause tau to become misshapen and toxic and to accumulate abnormally. Consequently, messages get off track, causing "train wrecks" in the brain that become toxic dumps, then larger trash piles known as neurofibrillary tangles. Normal neurotransmitter traffic can't get past the roadblocks; their communications shut off, the distressed neurons eventually die.

What to do? Focus on known ways to deplete these brain toxins and prevent their formation. Get enough sleep; going sleepless raises beta-amyloid levels. Controlling blood sugar, lowering insulin, losing weight, and treating diabetes all may lower beta-amyloid. DHA fish oil, caffeine, cinnamon, curcumin (in the spice turmeric), blueberries, boysenberries, cranberries, black currants, strawberries, dried plums, and grapes can reduce beta-amyloid in animal brains and in cell cultures.

Be on the alert for new discoveries about how to reduce, remove, or detoxify beta-amyloid and tau, slowing down their destruction of brain cells.

HAVE A **PURPOSE IN LIFE**

**Having a sense of direction and fulfillment
may keep you Alzheimer's-free**

D o you agree or disagree with these statements?
"I feel good when I think of what I have done in the past
and what I hope to do in the future."

"I have a sense of direction and purpose in life."

"I enjoy making plans for the future and working to make
them a reality."

"Some people wander aimlessly through life, but I am not
one of them."

If you strongly agree, you are likely to have a "greater purpose in life," which means you are about two and a half times
more likely to remain free of Alzheimer's than people who
have a gloomier, less fulfilled outlook on their lives. That's the
conclusion of a study that asked 951 people—average age
eighty, mostly women—to answer ten questions on a psychological test measuring overall sense of purpose in life. Initially
they were also tested cognitively; none had dementia.

Researchers at Rush University Medical Center and Rush Alzheimer's Disease Center in Chicago tracked the respondents for an average of four years. Sixteen percent of them developed Alzheimer's. The 10 percent who topped the purpose-in-life scale were most often spared. Those in the bottom 10 percent, with the least sense of purpose and fulfillment, were most likely to rapidly decline cognitively and be diagnosed with Alzheimer's.

The idea of having a greater purpose in life has a long history in psychology and according to researchers means "a tendency to derive meaning from life's experiences and to possess a sense of intentionality and goal directedness that guides behavior." This leads to a very personal feeling of well-being. It is independent of economic, job, and social success. A person making pies in a deli can have as great a sense of purpose as the CEO of a large corporation.

How does having a purposeful life translate into protection from the massive destruction of brain cells known as Alzheimer's? Interestingly, there may be a biological connection. Previous research at the University of Wisconsin, Madison, shows that people who rank high on "purpose in life" measures have lower blood levels of inflammatory and stress agents, higher good type HDL cholesterol, and a smaller waist-to-hip ratio! All are known to lower Alzheimer's risk. Rush University researchers also found that those with a strong life purpose lived longer and aged more successfully.

What to do? Since having a greater purpose in life is not a fixed personality trait, even small things you do can make it come alive, says Rush University investigator Aron S. Buchman, MD. Mainly, get involved in a way that you believe can make a difference. Volunteering is a powerful way to boost your sense of life purpose, studies show. So is having a part-time job if you are retired. Get and stay engaged with civic organizations and projects that make you feel needed and useful.

"Being useful to others instills a sense of being needed and valued," researchers report. Become and stay socially, physically, and mentally active. Make plans and set goals, and make them a reality. For example, make your own action plan to avoid Alzheimer's. (See "Putting It All Together," page 285.)

GET A GOOD NIGHT'S **SLEEP**

A lack of sleep is toxic to brain cells

Sleep has surprising powers to protect your brain against memory loss and Alzheimer's. In fact, skimping on sleep may trigger Alzheimer's-type brain damage. That mind-boggling discovery comes from recent research at Washington University Medical Center in Saint Louis.

In truth, sleep appears to be somewhat of a wonder drug. Its newly revealed secret: it helps manipulate levels of the dreaded peptide beta-amyloid, a prime instigator of Alzheimer's.

Keeping levels of this toxin lower by getting enough sleep in midlife might help prevent Alzheimer's symptoms years later, suspects David Holtzman, MD, head of neurology at Washington University. In an effort to understand sleep's effects on beta-amyloid, he enlisted mice genetically prone to Alzheimer's for a series of sleep tests. The results were dramatic. When the mice slept normally, their brain levels of toxic beta-amyloid went down about 25 percent. When they were awake, beta-amyloid levels went up.

Especially alarming for millions of sleep-deprived Americans is what happened to Holtzman's mice when they were forced to stay awake for long periods. Beta-amyloid deposits soared in the brains of mice that were nudged and dumped into water to keep them awake twenty hours a day. Further, Holtzman says he was astounded by the sharp rise in beta-amyloid plaques in the brains of sleep-starved mice compared with those allowed to snooze without interruption. No question, sleep deprivation accelerated the pathology of Alzheimer's.

Does this happen in humans? Yes, says Holtzman, beta-amyloid levels in cerebrospinal fluid go down when we sleep and rise when we are awake. It is reasonable to think, he speculates, that chronic exposure to abnormally high beta amyloid produced during sleep deprivation inflicts similar punishment on human brain cells.

Further, research at Wake Forest University School of Medicine finds that sleeping on average five hours or less a night is linked to large increases in dangerous visceral, or abdominal, fat, which can lead to obesity, insulin resistance, and diabetes, all of which raise your risk of dementia. In fact, only one sleepless night (four hours instead of the usual eight) induced insulin resistance in normal, healthy people, reported a recent Dutch study.

What to do? Don't think of sleep as an inconvenience but as a legitimate way to subdue some of the brain's most devastating enemies. Take naps. Seek treatment for sleep disorders, including sleep apnea and insomnia. Look for sleep clinics in your area. It's okay to miss your zzzz's sometimes. But chronic lack of sleep (less than the average six to eight hours daily for most adults) may have more serious consequences over the long term than you ever dreamed. Sleep on it.

81

FORGET ABOUT **SMOKING**

Smoking can steal years of good memory

Don't be surprised if that haze of cigarette smoke around your head gives you a hazy memory... or worse. Smoking nearly doubles your risk of developing Alzheimer's, according to a recent analysis of forty-three studies by researchers at the University of California, San Francisco.

Generally, the more you smoke, the quicker you may find yourself with both mild memory impairment and outright Alzheimer's. UCLA researchers have found that smoking more than a pack a day pushes you two to three years closer to Alzheimer's. If you have a history of heavy smoking and heavy drinking and a genetic risk (you carry the ApoE4 gene), you can expect to confront Alzheimer's *ten years earlier* than people with none of these risks.

Passive smoking can also ruin memory. Inhaling other people's smoke boosts the likelihood of memory problems by

44 percent, compared to avoiding smoke exposure, according to British investigators.

It's understandable: smoke infuses the brain with so-called free radicals, which, research shows, directly damage the cerebral cortex. Smoke also incites inflammation, another culprit in neurodegeneration. And don't forget: smoking can bring on strokes.

So, what about that widely believed odd idea that smoking can actually help prevent Alzheimer's? The truth is a few studies have shown that. But when University of California, San Francisco, researcher Janine Caltado, PhD, looked more closely at the data, she found that *only* studies done by researchers with ties to the tobacco industry found anti-Alzheimer's benefits from smoking. The studies without tobacco industry connections found a decided doubling of Alzheimer's risk if you smoke.

What to do? Try everything to kick the habit. The sooner you stop bathing your brain in clouds of smoke, the better your chances of fending off memory decline and possibly Alzheimer's, as well as cancer, cardiovascular disease, and strokes.

But there may be something to the idea that nicotine alone, stripped of the hazard of smoke, can have anti-Alzheimer's activity. Researchers are investigating the potential benefits by using skin patches to deliver nicotine to the brain, while eliminating the hazards from smoke. (See "Think About a Nicotine Patch," page 209.)

HAVE A BIG **SOCIAL CIRCLE**

Lots of friends and family can override
brain pathology

Imagine looking at the brain tissue of two different women under a microscope. One died at age eighty, the other at age ninety. Both had severe brain pathology— a mess of so-called "plaques and tangles" that confirmed a diagnosis of Alzheimer's. Yet in life, one acted like a person with Alzheimer's, while the other's mental functioning was so normal that doctors examining her ravaged brain could hardly believe it.

The intellectually intact woman had an extended circle of family and friends, explain researchers at Rush University Medical Center in Chicago. Her large social network gave her a strong "cognitive reserve" that enabled her to withstand the terrible devastation in her brain. Incredible as this all sounds, intimate social contacts help build a brain that seems somewhat oblivious to the accumulating destruction. "The pathology moves along at its own pace, but you don't lose your memory," says chief Alzheimer's researcher David Bennett, MD, of Rush University.

In fact, the ninety-year-old woman whose brain did not know she had Alzheimer's had a social network ten times larger than that of the younger woman who personified the disease. Despite the similar severity of brain plaques and tangles, the more socially active woman had recently scored much higher on tests of cognitive function than the more socially isolated woman.

It gets even more intriguing. The worse the physical degeneration of your brain, the more your intellect and memory benefit from interacting with a large circle of friends and family.

How an obviously deluded brain performs this miracle of making you seem mentally normal just because you keep lots of people close to you is a mystery. The best answer investigators can come up with, says Bennett, is that socializing makes the brain more efficient, prodding it to find new, alternative routes of communication to bypass piles of neuronal trash and broken connections left by Alzheimer's march through the brain. The stronger the brain reserve you build throughout life, the more likely you are to stave off Alzheimer's symptoms. (See "Build 'Cognitive Reserve,'" page 77.)

What to do? See old friends and family often, including not just your spouse and/or your children, but also grandchildren, nephews, nieces, uncles, aunts, cousins, in-laws—anyone you feel relatively close to or can talk to comfortably. Expand your social network; make new friends. What's important is regular contact—a feeling of being connected rather than isolated and lonely.

83

DON'T FORGET YOUR **SPINACH**

Leafy and cruciferous vegetables slow and reverse memory loss

Eating vegetables of all kinds does wonders to preserve your memory as you age. Being a vegetable lover cut rates of cognitive decline by up to 40 percent in a large group of older Americans studied at Chicago's Rush University. That means, says study author Martha Clare Morris, ScD, that eating 2.8 servings of vegetables a day, compared to less than 1 serving, could shave about five years off your cognitive age.

In a Harvard University study of more than thirteen thousand women, the most prodigious vegetable eaters had a slower rate of cognitive decline as they got older than the skimpiest vegetable eaters. The greatest protection came from two families of vegetables: leafy greens, such as spinach and lettuce, and cruciferous vegetables, including broccoli, Brussels sprouts, kale, cauliflower, and cabbage.

Neuroscientist James Joseph, PhD, at Tufts University,

became convinced of the power of spinach after witnessing its astonishing effects on the brains of lab animals. He started feeding spinach to rats early in life—comparable to age twenty in humans. No question: compared to non-spinach-eating rats, the spinach-fed animals had superior long-term memory, better learning ability, and far less brain damage at midlife and in old age. Spinach had prevented the expected age-related cognitive loss.

Then Joseph starting feeding rats spinach only *after* they got old—between ages sixty-five and seventy in human terms. They already had age-related diminished memory and brain deficits. Remarkably, the spinach rejuvenated their memory and learning ability back to "middle age," and their brain deficits regressed, too. Just think of it, marveled Joseph: spinach actually "fixed" their aged brains, reversing months of aging.

How much spinach? The equivalent of a large bowl of fresh spinach leaves a day. (Blueberries and strawberries had similar benefits; see "Eat Berries Every Day," page 43.)

Researchers mostly credit high antioxidants in deeply colored vegetables and fruits with fending off and repairing brain cell damage. Test-tube studies at Cornell University, for example, found red cabbage more effective than white in reducing the toxicity of beta-amyloid in brain cells, a telltale sign of Alzheimer's.

What to do? Eat vegetables—especially deep green, yellow, and red ones—with a passion. (White potatoes don't count.)

At least three servings — even better, five to nine servings — a day may help keep your aging memory intact and ward off Alzheimer's. Never pass up a chance to eat a colorful vegetable. The antioxidants in a vegetable here and there over many years can add up to significant brain protection.

INVESTIGATE **STATINS**

Do they prevent or help cause
memory problems?

Prescription drugs known as statins lower bad type LDL cholesterol and help tame inflammation, both factors implicated in Alzheimer's. That spurred hopes that statins might help prevent Alzheimer's. But despite early optimistic findings, the evidence argues otherwise, and some doctors report statins can even lead to memory problems.

It sounds "intuitive" that statins should work, says one expert. People with high cholesterol in midlife are more apt to develop Alzheimer's, and Alzheimer's patients often have high cholesterol. Still, study after study found no brain protection from taking statins. Among a group of elderly nuns, for example, taking statins had no impact on their risk of Alzheimer's, cognitive decline, or pathologic brain changes indicative of Alzheimer's, according to Rush University researchers.

Most convincing is a major 2009 review by the Cochrane Collaboration, an international organization that evaluates medical research. Investigators looked at the use of two statins, Zocor and Pravachol, in double-blind controlled studies involving 26,340 patients at high risk of dementia and Alzheimer's. The clear message: there was no difference in the incidence of dementia or cognitive status among older people who took the cholesterol-lowering drugs for up to five years.

This "gold-standard" double-blind controlled test, says study author Bernadette McGuinness, MD, at Queen's University in Belfast, Ireland, is compelling evidence that taking statins late in life does *not* protect against dementia. She says she doesn't know whether taking statins in *midlife* for many years might stave off dementia later in life. Studies to answer that question have not been done.

Statins also flunked as an enhancer of cognitive function among ordinary older people not highly prone to Alzheimer's. An older group in Spain who took various statins (Mevacor, Altocor, Zocor, Lipitor, Lescol, Pravachol) for two years did no better on cognitive and memory tests than a control group of non–statin takers, according to researchers at Columbia University's College of Physicians and Surgeons.

Thus, no current evidence exists that statins boost memory or prevent cognitive decline and Alzheimer's in older people. Whether statins could be detrimental, especially in late life, is also unanswered.

The Cochrane study did not find cognitive harm from statins. However, the possibility is increasingly controversial. Many anecdotal reports and some studies reveal memory disturbances in people who take statins. Beatrice Golomb, MD, at the University of California, San Diego, School of Medicine, keeps track of adverse effects of statins. Her recent analysis found that "cognitive problems" are second only to muscle problems in statin takers but are rarely recognized by prescribing doctors.

What to do? If you take statins for cardiovascular reasons, continue under your doctor's direction and monitoring. But don't count on statins to prevent or delay the onset or progression of cognitive impairment or Alzheimer's. If you notice side effects from cholesterol-lowering statins, report them to your doctor. You can also read about and report adverse effects at Golomb's website, www.statinstudy@ucsd.edu.

85

SURROUND YOURSELF WITH **STIMULATION**

A socially, physically, and mentally rich environment discourages Alzheimer's

Thank heaven for scientists who like to see little animals thrive. Otherwise, how could we know our aging brains flourish when surrounded by social, physical, and mental stimulation? It's impossible to do huge studies over the lifetime of people to find this out. So scientists use lab animals as stand-ins to test whether living in an "enriched environment" discourages brain degeneration.

A pioneer in the study of this phenomenon is William Greenough, PhD, a neuroscientist at the University of Illinois at Urbana-Champaign. He built a cage he called "a Disneyland for rats," with toys, running wheels, hidden food, obstacles, and lots of companion rats. For comparison, he housed other rats, alone or in pairs, in bleak cages.

Greenough then examined the animals' brains. The residents of "Disneyland," including old rats, had brains lush with new growth—longer, more complex dendrites; more synapses; new blood vessels—and were smarter on cognitive tests than "the cage potatoes." He concluded that living in an enriched environment stimulates brains to grow stronger and be less vulnerable to age-related memory loss and Alzheimer's.

At the Alzheimer's Disease Research Center at the University of South Florida, researcher Gary Arendash, PhD, takes the idea further. He tries to figure out which type of stimulation— social, physical, or mental—is most brain protective. He, too, set up mice to live either isolated in an "impoverished environment" or with playmates in fun houses with extravagant amusements and activities—"an enriched environment." His key finding: mice exposed to intellectual, physical, and social stimulation had lower amounts of toxic beta-amyloid (a hallmark of Alzheimer's) in their brains. But beta-amyloid did not diminish in animals engaged only in physical and/or social activities. Thus, Arendash says, mental stimulation appears more powerful than other activities in fending off Alzheimer's, although being social and exercising contribute to protection.

An intriguing study at Sweden's Karolinska Institute agrees that all three types of stimulation pay off big-time—and are better than one or two activities alone. Researchers asked 776 men and women over age seventy-five how often they participated in twenty-nine activities, including reading, going to theaters and museums, walking, playing bingo, singing, engaging in politics, meeting friends, and doing sports. Then researchers teased out the mental, physical, and social components of each activity and added them up. Most apt to reduce the likelihood of dementia six years later was being social, followed by being physically active, and then mentally active. However, people who scored highest in all three categories— mental, physical, and social—were least apt to end up with dementia; their risk dropped by half. Bottom line: your brain thrives best on a wide variety of mental, physical, and social stimulation.

What to do? Surround yourself with an environment that is intellectually, physically, and socially stimulating. That may include lots of friends and relatives, books or electronic reading material, a computer, a telescope, musical instruments, sculpture, paintings, needlepoint, board games, cards, jigsaw puzzles, Wii games, a digital camera, a video camera, gardening, a treadmill, a swimming pool, a pool table, table tennis— whatever attracts you. Make it a rich and ever-changing playground. Bringing in new "toys" and experiences helps keep the neurons in your brain alert, frisky, efficient, and alive—with increased fortitude against the threat of a declining memory and Alzheimer's. (See "Do Something New," page 203, and "Build 'Cognitive Reserve,'" page 77.)

86

DEAL WITH **STRESS**

It puts unwanted hormones in your brain

When you are under stress, your body pours out hormones called corticosteroids, including cortisol. This stress reaction and consequent surge of adrenaline can save you in a crisis. But persistent stress reactions, triggered by everyday events such as work frustration, traffic jams, and financial worries, keep your brain bathed in cortisol. And that's dangerous. Over time, it can destroy brain cells and suppress the growth of new ones, actually shrinking your brain.

Researchers at McGill University in Montreal followed fifty older people for more than fifteen years, comparing cortisol levels with memory decline. Those whose cortisol progressively increased to high levels had more memory impairment than those with moderate cortisol levels. The hippocampus—a memory region of the brain—also was about 14 percent smaller in the stressed-out high-cortisol people. The blame, researchers concluded, was prolonged cortisol exposure that probably led to irreversible brain damage. One woman with high cortisol who developed depression and Alzheimer's lost about 60 percent of her total brain volume within five years.

Moreover, sudden traumatic events can leave a hangover of severe psychological stress that precedes dementia. Greek neurologists at Aristotle University of Thessaloniki tell of a forty-nine-year-old woman who was diagnosed with dementia after the death of her father. And of a man who started deteriorating mentally after losing all his property; he was later diagnosed with Alzheimer's. Others have noted the onset of dementia soon after the loss of a loved one or a life-changing event such as retirement.

Older veterans with post-traumatic stress disorder (PTSD) are nearly twice as likely to develop dementia as veterans without the disorder, according to research at the University of California, San Francisco. "It's not surprising," says Robert S. Wilson, PhD, a neuropsychologist at the Rush Alzheimer's Disease Center in Chicago. He points out that although PTSD may not directly cause dementia, it may make people more vulnerable to it.

What to do? Be aware that chronic stress and PTSD can hike older people's vulnerability to memory decline and dementia. Seek professional advice. Antidepressants, counseling, relaxation techniques, and other forms of therapy may head off stress-related memory loss if it is noticed and treated in the early stages. In a recent University of Connecticut survey, 66 percent of the public did not know that high stress is a risk factor for dementia.

87

AVOID **STROKES**

A stroke doubles your odds of Alzheimer's

A stroke is a vascular accident that you want to avoid for two important reasons: it brings its own specific damage, and it sets you up for Alzheimer's. In fact, even if your brain has some Alzheimer's pathology, symptoms may not appear unless a stroke comes along to flip the switch and cause enough additional damage to trigger dementia. A full-blown stroke at least doubles your chances of developing Alzheimer's.

In some cases, even small strokes in strategic parts of the brain can hike your risk of Alzheimer's by a staggering twenty times, according to landmark findings by noted brain researcher David Snowdon, PhD, at the University of Kentucky. Stroke damage on top of Alzheimer's plaques and tangles brings worse brain devastation than either condition alone. As Snowdon said, "Stroke plus Alzheimer's is not one plus one equals two. It's more like one plus one equals four or five."

Why? For one thing, researchers know that after a stroke,

the brain shows increased production of toxic beta-amyloid, the sticky gunk that sets off Alzheimer's. Columbia University investigators speculate that the beta-amyloid is stimulated by a specific protein that is released in the aftermath of a stroke. Strokes are also accompanied by inflammation, another prominent villain in Alzheimer's.

Strokes, especially ministrokes, are also a prime cause of vascular dementia, a disease of the brain's blood vessels and capillaries that has symptoms similar to Alzheimer's. The two diseases often occur in the brain simultaneously. (See "Prevent Vascular Dementia," page 264.)

What to do? Keep blood pressure down; high blood pressure is the number-one cause of strokes. (See "Control Blood Pressure," page 49.) Stop smoking; this reduces stroke risk dramatically. Exercise; in a recent study, older men who got moderate to heavy exercise were 63 percent less apt to have a stroke. Eat lots of fruits and vegetables for a high intake of potassium, a known stroke deterrent. Take vitamin D; people with very low vitamin D levels are 78 percent more apt to have a stroke than those with normal vitamin D. Watch for early signs of stroke risk; have your carotid (neck) arteries checked by ultrasound to detect any blockage that could cut off blood to your brain. Also have your ankle blood pressure checked. (See "Check Out Your Ankle," page 24.)

CUT DOWN ON **SUGAR**

Too much creates Alzheimer's plaques
in the brain

Feeding your brain too much sugar is a huge mistake. Here's what happened to Alzheimer's-prone mice given drinking water spiked with 10 percent table sugar (sucrose), along with a "balanced diet," for most of their adult lives: they got fat and had high cholesterol and ineffectual insulin. On learning and memory tests they were duds. The clincher: their brains, compared to those of mice given plain water, contained *three times as much* beta-amyloid, that sticky gunk that kills neurons and initiates Alzheimer's.

Yes, the sobering fact is that ordinary sugar spurs production of the toxic stuff that leads to Alzheimer's in susceptible brains. How much sugar did the brain-damaged mice drink? The human equivalent of forty teaspoons of sugar (six hundred calories) a day, according to researchers at the University of Alabama at Birmingham. "It may take less to cause similar damage in humans," they added.

And pity the poor laboratory rats that gorge directly on fructose, as in high-fructose corn syrup, commonly used to sweeten soft drinks and processed foods. Researchers at Georgia State University have vividly described how such animals, after learning something, cannot remember it the next day. They flail around in water, searching for a safe platform to swim to, clueless as to where it used to be. Their "spatial memory" is seriously impaired. Experts now say loss of spatial memory is an early sign of Alzheimer's in humans.

And if the direct brain damage from sugar hits is not scary enough, our longtime love affair with sugar also sparks our epidemic of obesity, diabetes, high blood pressure, high triglycerides, low HDL good cholesterol, and so-called metabolic syndrome, a combination of several risk factors. All of these are indirect highways to age-related memory impairment and Alzheimer's.

Worst is high-fructose corn syrup, because it creates the most vicious type of fat—visceral, or belly, fat that lies deep in the abdomen, forming a bulging "apple shape." Dramatic proof comes from a test at the University of California, Davis. Overweight and obese individuals drank special beverages spiked with either pure fructose or pure glucose. After ten weeks, their weight varied only slightly, but the fructose drinkers had piled on an astounding 80 percent more visceral fat. They also had higher fasting blood sugar, triglycerides, detrimental LDL cholesterol, and, worst of all, dysfunctional insulin, or "insulin resistance," which has direct ties to cognitive impairment and dementia. (See "Keep Insulin Normal," page 159, and "Watch Your Waist," page 276.)

Bottom line: eating plain sugar is bad enough in promoting Alzheimer's, but loading up on high-fructose processed foods and beverages dramatically multiplies the threat.

What to do? Make a conscious effort to cut back on sugar of all types. Don't drink obesity-generating sugary soft drinks; a twelve-ounce can has eight teaspoons of sugar, usually high-fructose corn syrup. Depend mostly on fruits and other natural sources for sweeteners. (Fructose as it comes in fruits is okay.) Check the labels of processed foods for added and hidden sugars, such as corn sweetener, corn syrup, dextrose, glucose, high-fructose corn syrup, honey, maltose, malt syrup, molasses, sucrose, and syrup.

Listen to the American Heart Association: it advises most women to limit added sugar in foods and drinks to six teaspoons (100 calories) a day, and most men to nine teaspoons (150 calories) a day. Replace sugary soft drinks with plain or carbonated water, unsweetened iced tea, juices, low-fat milk, and occasional artificially sweetened soft drinks.

89

DRINK **TEA**

It may block strokes and memory loss and revive dying neurons

Researchers have discovered fascinating ways common tea can save your brain from dementia. The latest "exciting findings," as described by researchers at UCLA: If you drink at least three cups of green or black tea a day, your likelihood of having a stroke drops 21 percent. And if you double the intake, your stroke probability falls 42 percent. Admittedly, that's a monumental promise from such a small gesture.

And the most compelling news: much evidence suggests that tea stalls the cognitive loss that precedes Alzheimer's dementia and that the more tea you drink, the sharper your aging memory is. Elderly Japanese men and women who drank only a cup of green tea a day cut their odds of cognitive impairment 38 percent. Older Americans who drink black or green tea only once to four times a week have 37 percent less cognitive decline annually than non-tea drinkers, finds new UCLA research.

Tea's secret is no mystery. The leaves are packed with

compounds able to penetrate the blood-brain barrier and block neuronal damage. Lab rats raised on green tea, for example, have less damage in the hippocampus, or memory processing region of the brain, and consequently have vastly superior memories and learning abilities in old age.

One particularly powerful green tea antioxidant, EGCG (epigallocatechin-3-gallate), can block the toxicity of beta-amyloid, which kills brain cells, and remove, or "chelate," destructive iron from the brain. In groundbreaking experiments, Israeli scientists found that EGCG can even revive sick and dying neurons thought lost to degenerative brain disease. Bringing back withered brain cells from the brink of death to robust life is big-time help for anybody's brain.

What to do? Make it a point to drink real, *brewed* black and green tea (*Camellia sinensis*). Both benefit your aging brain, although green tea has three to four times more antioxidants, notably high doses of EGCG. Instant, bottled, or canned "real" teas, as well as herbal teas, have little antioxidant activity. To extract the most antioxidants, let the tea bag or loose tea steep in hot water for at least five minutes. Don't add milk; it can reduce tea's antioxidant activity by as much as 25 percent.

For extra brain protection, you can take green tea extracts that deliver high doses of EGCG, available at health food stores or drugstores and online. Israeli investigators say that 300 to 400 mg of straight EGCG in supplement form is an adequate dose.

90

TAKE CARE OF YOUR **TEETH**

Bad gums may poison your brain

People with tooth and gum disease are apt to score lower on memory and cognition tests, according to a University of West Virginia School of Dentistry analysis. Researcher Richard Crout, DDS, theorizes that an infection responsible for gum disease gives off inflammatory by-products that travel to areas of the brain involved in memory loss. These inflammatory agents may be toxic to brain cells. Consequently, Crout says brushing, flossing, and generally preventing gum disease may help keep your gums and teeth healthy, and also your memory sharper.

Research at the University of Southern California comparing pairs of twins found that having periodontal disease, characterized by loose and missing teeth, before age thirty-five quadrupled the likelihood of having dementia later in life. The probable culprit: a lifetime exposure to inflammation that not only weakens gum structure but also harms brain tissue.

Older Americans with the most severe gingivitis—inflamed gums, a first sign of periodontal disease—are two to three times more likely to show signs of impaired memory and cognition than those with the least gingivitis, according to neurologists at Columbia University's College of Physicians and Surgeons.

What to do? Be sure you and everyone in your family get treatment early in life to control bleeding, inflamed gums. It could help save your brain from inflammatory assaults leading to memory loss and dementia later in life, experts say.

91

HAVE YOUR **THYROID** CHECKED

Overactive or sluggish, it could bring on Alzheimer's

A faulty thyroid can mimic the symptoms of Alzheimer's. That's why a dysfunctional thyroid can lead to a misdiagnosis of dementia. Happily, drugs usually correct the problem and the faux dementia vanishes.

But now there's new reason to worry about your thyroid. Abnormal thyroid activity might actually bring on Alzheimer's. In fact, if you are a woman, thyroid problems double your odds of developing Alzheimer's, according to recent research.

Zaldy S. Tan, MD, and colleagues at Harvard Medical School and Boston University School of Medicine followed more than eighteen hundred men and women, average age seventy-one, for about thirteen years. At the beginning of the study, all were cognitively intact; at the end, about 11 percent had been diagnosed with Alzheimer's.

Women who were either hypothyroid or hyperthyroid — with the lowest and highest blood levels of thyroid-stimulating hormone (TSH) — had twice the rate of Alzheimer's as women with normal levels. Interestingly, this study showed that men with abnormal thyroid were not more likely to get Alzheimer's. However, in subsequent Dutch research, older men who were hyperthyroid did have a 20 percent jump in Alzheimer's risk over normal or hypothyroid men.

How could thyroid dysfunction lead to Alzheimer's? Researchers suggest some possible reasons: Excessive thyroid hormone may kill neurons and deplete the neurotransmitter acetylcholine or damage cerebral blood vessels. Low thyroid may increase toxic beta-amyloid in brain cells.

What to do? If you suspect thyroid problems, get a routine thyroid test. If you have been diagnosed with Alzheimer's, get a thyroid test to rule out a misdiagnosis. In the Harvard–Boston University study, people with increased Alzheimer's risk had TSH levels under 1.0 or over 2.10; researchers say that these levels identify more people as abnormal than standard guidelines do. Thyroid problems can usually be corrected by medication.

Symptoms of thyroid problems are many, but common signs of an underactive thyroid include fatigue, depression, and weight gain. Signs of an overactive thyroid are irritability, weight loss, increased resting pulse rate, muscle weakness, a fine tremor in the hands, and insomnia. Cognitive decline may be a symptom of both underactive and overactive thyroids.

92

BEWARE OF BEING **UNDERWEIGHT**

Dropping pounds late in life may signal Alzheimer's

Although middle-age obesity ups your odds of Alzheimer's, unexplained weight loss after age sixty or so may be a sign of Alzheimer's in your future.

Mayo Clinic investigators noted that women started losing weight at least ten years before dementia was diagnosed. Among women of equal weight (140 pounds on average), those who went on to develop dementia slowly became thinner over three decades and, when diagnosed, weighed an average twelve pounds less than women who were free of Alzheimer's. Weight among those destined for Alzheimer's fell to 136 pounds ten years before the onset of symptoms and to 128 pounds by the time of diagnosis. Weight among women without dementia was steady over the same period.

Apparently, the weight loss is spurred by early brain pathology rather than by an eating disorder or restriction in food intake due to cognitive changes, says James Mortimer, PhD, at the University of South Florida. His study of elderly women discovered that unexplained weight loss was mirrored by severe brain deterioration. "Given its very long duration prior to onset of dementia, it is likely that weight loss is specifically associated with the Alzheimer disease process," he concluded.

As brain pathology progresses, the rate of weight loss picks up, doubling in the year before symptoms are detectable, another study at Washington University found. And sudden unintentional weight loss in your seventies can triple your chances of developing dementia, according to research by Tiffany Hughes, PhD, at the University of Pittsburgh School of Medicine. The odds are even worse if you are overweight or obese to start with. That doesn't mean staying fat is good for you, she says. It's just that sudden weight loss later in life may be a warning sign of approaching dementia before the disease symptoms become evident.

Bottom line: obesity in middle age may be a risk factor for dementia, while declining weight in late life may reflect brain changes predictive of Alzheimer's. Leading authority Rachel A. Whitmer, PhD, at Kaiser Permanente's Division of Research, says that a body-mass index (BMI) of under 18.5 in an elderly person is a risk factor for Alzheimer's.

What to do? Since gradual or steep unintentional weight loss may be tied to ongoing brain pathology, it is something to be watched and not necessarily regarded as a sign of health. You should investigate. Talk with your doctor about any unexplained weight loss after age sixty.

Should you deliberately try to lose weight in late life? The standard advice from some doctors and researchers has been no. They worry that weight loss could lead to frailty or earlier death, as some studies have concluded. However, Wake Forest University research recently found that overweight elderly people who *intentionally* lost weight (an average of ten pounds) by exercising had a 50 percent lower risk of death over the next eight years. Such findings support sensible weight loss even in old age. But don't overdo it. Frailty (weight loss, especially from muscle mass; poor grip strength; slower walking; a drop in overall physical activity; and exhaustion) in the elderly is a huge risk factor for rapid cognitive decline.

PREVENT **VASCULAR DEMENTIA**

Tiny injuries in your brain's blood vessels steal your mind

Alzheimer's jumps to mind when you think of dementia, and indeed it is the number one cause of dementia. But second, and equally destructive to an aging brain, is vascular dementia.

Researchers used to think the two dementias were totally separate, but now say they are closely related. About 50 percent of people with Alzheimer's pathology also have severe brain blood vessel damage. Since the symptoms of both dementias are extremely similar, doctors have a hard time telling them apart, and even more so when they exist simultaneously and the symptoms are multiplied. Vascular dementia is frequently misdiagnosed as Alzheimer's. Although the two dementias feed on each other, they mainly arise from different brain problems.

Vascular dementia happens because blood flow in the brain is reduced or blocked, leaving neurons to starve and die. The primary cause of restricted blood flow or blockage is accumulated damage to cerebral vessels from strokes—either a major stroke or, more typically, multiple ministrokes, also called silent strokes, because they go unnoticed. Very early predictors of memory impairment show up on MRI brain scans as white spots known as "white matter hyperintensities," which are associated with high blood pressure. Another telltale sign of vascular dementia is difficulty with balance and walking. The underlying reasons for vascular dementia are cardiovascular, including high blood pressure, high cholesterol, hardening of the arteries, inflammation, and diabetes.

A primary difference between vascular dementia and Alzheimer's is disease progression. In Alzheimer's, cognitive decline is slow, steady, and rather consistent. In vascular dementia, cognition can decline abruptly as cells die off from repeated ministrokes or even major strokes. The good news about vascular dementia is that although the damage appears irreversible, preventing further strokes helps stop the cognitive decline.

What to do? Do everything you can to prevent damage to blood vessels in your brain. That means keeping blood pressure normal (blood pressure is the major cause of strokes) and reducing cholesterol and inflammation (which damage brain capillaries). Be on the alert for a deficiency of vitamin B_{12}, which can lead to increased white matter hyperintensities—an early sign of future vascular dementia. (See "Control Blood Pressure," page 49, "Control Bad Cholesterol," page 66, and "Fight Inflammation," page 153.)

94

PLAY VIDEO GAMES

They may improve memory and reaction times, which decline with age

What happens when older people start playing video games? Well, it depends on the game, but Arthur Kramer, PhD, an eminent researcher and a psychology professor at the University of Illinois at Urbana-Champaign, has good news. In a recent test, he recruited an over-sixty group to play a computer game called Rise of Nations for eight weeks to see if it boosted their cognitive skills. This particular video game is a complex, strategy-based role-playing game in which players build their own empires. That means planning cities, feeding and employing people, and maintaining an adequate military, all of which requires lots of decision making and multitasking.

Remember, the gamers were novices; they had played zero video games in the previous two years. So Kramer knew it would mean nothing much if they simply learned to play the game better over time, which they did. What he wanted to know was whether playing Rise of Nations lifted their cognitive functioning generally. If so, it would mean the video game provided the type of mental stimulation that can delay or reverse age-related cognitive losses.

To Kramer's delight, after eight weeks, the practice the gamers got did enable them to score higher on tests of "executive control"—including task switching, working memory, visual short-term memory, and reasoning—than oldsters who had not played the game. These are precisely the cognitive abilities most impaired in people over sixty. Interestingly, playing the game did nothing for the cognition of college students in their early twenties. The game apparently worked because it targeted mental skills that had diminished in older people.

This experiment is the first of its kind to provide evidence that complex intellect-engaging video games can counter the loss of cognitive functioning in late life.

What about playing simplistic action video games, such as God of War, that require rapid information processing and quick reactions? A study at the University of Rochester in New York suggests that such fast-paced video games could markedly improve older people's reaction times and speed of processing information and contribute to enhancing memory and spatial reasoning. There's good evidence that "the very act of playing action video games significantly reduces reaction times," according to the study.

What to do? Go ahead—have fun with video games, including the popular Wii games (virtual bowling, tennis, golf, and boxing, as well as an exercise fitness program). If you enjoy action video games, try those, too. And for a real challenge, take on intricate games like Rise of Nations. Kramer says there's no guarantee that all video games will make you smarter or better able to resist Alzheimer's. On the other hand, if a game is mentally stimulating and enjoyable, chances are it's good for your brain. And for mental stimulation, it's likely to beat watching television. (See "Google Something," page 132.)

95

PUT **VINEGAR** IN EVERYTHING

It helps control blood sugar and appetite

Don't expect vinegar to confront Alzheimer's directly. But there is plenty of evidence that vinegar sinks risk factors that may lead to memory decline and dementia—namely, high blood sugar, insulin resistance, diabetes and prediabetes, and weight gain. World-class researchers take vinegar very seriously.

What we need is a simple, effective way to lower blood glucose, says S. Mitchell Harman, MD, at the Kronos Longevity Research Institute in Phoenix. What comes to mind? Vinegar, he says, noting that studies in humans and animals show that the acidic stuff packs potent glucose-lowering effects. His institute is doing rigorous tests to find out precisely why it works.

Jennie Brand-Miller, PhD, a professor at the University of Sydney in Australia and a driving force behind the low-glycemic index diet, praises vinegar for putting the lid on foods that spike blood sugar. She says that four teaspoons of vinegar in your salad dressing can lower blood sugar spikes from an average meal by 30 percent. Putting vinegar on blood-sugar-hiking white potatoes can reduce surges by 25 percent. And downing two tablespoons of vinegar before you go to bed at night, Brand-Miller says, can help ensure lower blood sugar when you wake up in the morning, especially in diabetics.

Vinegar works, she theorizes, by putting the brakes on stomach emptying, slowing the digestion of carbs and possibly dampening appetite.

Studies at Arizona State University have found that vinegar can curb appetite and food intake, helping prevent weight gain and obesity, which are associated with diabetes, accelerated dementia, and memory loss. Subjects who took one and a half tablespoons of apple cider vinegar ate two hundred fewer calories at the next meal.

Swedish investigators agree. In one study, downing two or three tablespoons of vinegar with white bread cut expected rises in insulin and blood sugar by about 25 percent. The subjects also felt fuller; satiety is another key to vinegar's success.

What to do? Pour on the vinegar—add it to salad dressings, eat it by the spoonful, even mix it into a glass of drinking water. Any type of vinegar works—apple cider, white, balsamic, red wine, white wine, rice, raspberry, blueberry, and other fruit-flavored varieties—because it's the acidity that counts. Yes, that means that lemon and lime juice also help curb blood sugar rises, says Brand-Miller.

96

GET ENOUGH **VITAMIN B$_{12}$**

A lack of B$_{12}$ shrinks your brain

As you age, blood levels of B$_{12}$ go down and the chances of Alzheimer's go up. Your ability to absorb B$_{12}$ from foods diminishes in middle age, setting the stage for brain degeneration years later. One study found that having low B$_{12}$ in midlife quadrupled your likelihood of Alzheimer's in late life.

Recently, British scientists at the University of Oxford discovered why a brain running low on B$_{12}$ may have cognitive failure: brain mass actually shrinks. Using MRI brain imaging, researcher Anna Vogiatzoglou studied more than one hundred volunteers ages sixty-one to eighty-seven. Her remarkable finding: over a five-year period, those lowest in B$_{12}$ experienced six times more brain shrinkage than those highest in B$_{12}$. Surprisingly, no subjects were overtly B$_{12}$ "deficient." Even having what doctors call "low-normal" B$_{12}$ was associated with some of the worst brain shrinkage. It's not unusual for people to be misdiagnosed with Alzheimer's when the real cause is a B_{12} deficiency.

Researchers say a shortage of B_{12} causes brain atrophy by ripping away myelin, a fatty protective sheath around neurons. Also, a lack of B_{12} can trigger inflammation, another destroyer of brain cells. Low B_{12} also contributes to high levels of homocysteine, an amino acid incriminated in Alzheimer's.

What to do? Take 500 to 1,000 mcg of vitamin B_{12} daily after age forty. It is inexpensive and utterly safe; no side effects or toxic doses of B_{12} have been found. If you or an older family member has unexplained confusion, memory loss, fatigue, or signs of dementia, be sure to get tested for B_{12} deficiency. Most doctors do it routinely. If you are deficient, your doctor may recommend biweekly or monthly B_{12} shots until your B_{12} is normalized. Research shows that taking B_{12} tablets (usually 1,000 mcg a day) can replace shots once adequate levels of B_{12} are restored. Be sure to take vitamin B_{12} too if you take folic acid. (See "Take Folic Acid," page 127, and "Keep Homocysteine Normal," page 144.)

97

DON'T NEGLECT **VITAMIN D**

A shortage can prime your brain for Alzheimer's

I f you are deficient in vitamin D, you are more likely to face cognitive impairment and Alzheimer's. That idea wasn't even on most researchers' radar a few years ago. But mounting evidence suggests it's true. It's also alarming, because vitamin D deficiency is a global epidemic. Experts estimate that from 40 to 100 percent of older adults in the United States and Europe are vitamin D deficient.

The likelihood of mental decline and dementia goes up as your vitamin D level goes down. A recent major study of 3,325 Americans over age sixty-five showed that being "deficient" in vitamin D raised the odds of cognitive impairment 42 percent, and being "severely deficient" boosted the odds 394 percent! Those with the highest blood levels of vitamin D had the lowest risk.

Further, most older Americans are low in vitamin D and fail to take adequate supplements, leaving them exceptionally vulnerable to cognitive deterioration and possible dementia, according to lead researcher David Llewellyn, PhD, at the University of Exeter in England.

Will getting your vitamin D up slow cognitive decline as you age? Clinical trials haven't been done to prove it. But researchers have every reason to believe that upping vitamin D intake will help ward off dementia and other factors, such as depression and cardiovascular disease, associated with dementia.

The most exciting evidence for how vitamin D might fight Alzheimer's comes from groundbreaking research at UCLA. It shows that vitamin D improves the ability of the immune system's cleanup crews to go into the brain and remove bits of beta-amyloid, sticky deposits blamed for Alzheimer's destruction of neurons. Vitamin D strengthens the ability of scavengers, called macrophages, to gobble up waste products, including beta-amyloid. Researchers call it "clearing the brain" of amyloid. It's a big deal, since experts believe that removing the toxin should help prevent brain cell injury and death, thereby slowing or even reversing memory loss and Alzheimer's.

What to do? Ask your doctor for a vitamin D test to check your serum level of 25-hydroxyvitamin D, especially if you are over sixty. Typically, you are not "deficient" if you have a level of 30 ng/mL or above. But many experts advocate a more optimal level of at least 50 to 60 ng/mL.

You can raise your vitamin D three ways. One, eat vitamin-D rich foods, such as fatty fish (especially salmon and tuna); also milk, breakfast cereals, and some orange juice brands that are fortified with vitamin D. Two, get some sun-light. Your body synthesizes vitamin D from exposure to sun, but aging reduces the benefits. Three, take supplements of vitamin D, preferably the more potent D_3 form.

There is no consensus on dose. Some experts recommend 1,000 to 2,000 IUs of vitamin D daily. Top researchers often take 5,000 IU daily, says Robert Heaney, MD, a vitamin D expert at Creighton University. Indeed, a recent study at the University of Saskatchewan, Canada, showed that older people required a 5,000 IU daily dose to avoid a vitamin D deficiency, but that younger people could get by with 2,000 IU. Officially, the safe upper dose of vitamin D is 2,000 IU daily, but unoffi-cially experts put it at 10,000 IU. Harvard Medical School researcher Eric Rimm, ScD, offers this rule of thumb: each 100 IU of vitamin D per day increases blood levels by 1 ng/mL; a blood level over 150 ng/mL is excessive. Consult your doctor about a recommended dose, depending on the results of your blood test and/or medical condition.

WATCH YOUR **WAIST**

It's not just fat but the fat around your middle that can lead to Alzheimer's

You may already know that being overweight can heighten your odds of Alzheimer's. But it's not that simple. After years of mystery, researchers have figured out that the major factor is not just how fat you are, but how much fat you carry around your waist. A potbelly or a big stomach—that is, abdominal fat, as determined by the circumference or diameter of your waist—rather than your total weight or BMI is the real villain in late-life brain breakdown. Further, it is this abdominal flab, also referred to as central or visceral obesity, in *midlife* that sets the stage for destructive happenings in your brain years later.

Here are the facts from prominent researcher Rachel A. Whitmer, PhD, at Kaiser Permanente's Division of Research in Oakland, California. She compared the waist measurements of 6,583 subjects, taken when they were ages forty to forty-five, with their mental acuity three decades later. Her conclusion:

men and women with the largest waists in middle age, compared to those with the slimmest, were *three times more likely to have dementia*. Even normal-weight people who had a big belly or an "apple shape" in midlife were twice as apt to develop dementia. Not surprisingly, most predictive of dementia was being both obese and having an oversized waist.

Now here's a paradox: if you are overweight and elderly, your risk of dementia may not increase but actually drop. That's because a strong predictor of Alzheimer's in late life is weight loss, usually five to ten years before symptoms are noticeable. Thus, being underweight in old age may be an early warning sign of Alzheimer's. (See "Beware of Being Underweight," page 261.)

Still, even in old age, a big stomach can be hazardous to your brain. A recent University of Michigan study of 1,351 people ages 60 to 101 sums it up this way: individuals who were fattest overall, compared to the thinnest, were surprisingly only half as likely to suffer cognitive decline and dementia. A striking exception was those with big bellies. They were nearly twice as likely to have cognitive impairment and dementia. The message: abdominal fat, even in old age, may still predict brain degeneration, whereas just being plain fat overall in your elder years may be neutral or brain protective.

Why? The probable culprit is visceral fat, which accumulates in the abdominal cavity. Such fat is biologically active and behaves like a gland to promote insulin resistance, high blood sugar, high blood pressure, low good HDL cholesterol, inflammation, and type 2 diabetes. A lifetime of exposure to such metabolic dysregulation induced by belly fat is primarily responsible for the increased risk of mental decline and dementia, says Whitmer. The larger your waist, the more visceral fat you have, and the worse your risk.

What to do? One way to curb abdominal fat is to lose weight: visceral fat seems to drop off first. (Caution: elderly people should not become underweight.) Avoid trans fats and high-fructose corn syrup: both promote belly fat. By far the best way to prevent and take off visceral belly fat is to exercise. To stop visceral fat from creeping on (as it typically does in sedentary people of middle age), do regular moderate exercise—a brisk half-hour walk six times a week prevented visceral fat buildup in middle-aged people in a Duke University study. To take off excess visceral fat, you need to do more vigorous aerobic exercise—probably an hour at least three times a week. Obese men on such an aerobic exercise regimen dropped 18 percent of their abdominal fat in three months. Don't count on spot exercises such as sit-ups to get rid of visceral fat.

99

WALK, WALK, WALK

A brisk daily walk is a huge boost for your brain

Of all the physical exercise you can give your brain, the easi- est is walking. Researchers praise it. According to leading authority Arthur Kramer, PhD, a neuroscientist at the Univer- sity of Illinois at Urbana-Champaign, six months of regular aerobic walking pays off with an astonishing 15 to 20 percent improvement in memory, decision-making ability, and atten- tion, plus a bigger brain with more gray matter.

That's what he found in his classic study of sixty- to eighty- year-olds who went from being sedentary to engaging in aero- bic exercise—mostly brisk walking on a treadmill for an hour at least three times a week. Older people in the study who merely stretched and toned did not derive cognitive benefits.

Most astonishing were MRI scans showing that brain vol- ume in the aerobic walkers had *increased,* notably in crucial areas of gray matter involved in the type of memory, learning, and thinking abilities that decline with age. Thus, aerobic walking was able not just to stall cognitive impairment but to actually *reverse* it by adding new brain mass. A bigger brain definitely translates into a better memory and cognitive functioning, says Kramer. In fact, after just six months of aerobic walking, the exercisers' brains looked two to three years younger on MRIs than they actually were, he noted. That probably means brain circuits work better because of new vascular structure, new neurons, and new neuronal connections created by walking, says Kramer.

He credits the incredible brain growth and improved cognitive functioning to the fact the once-sedentary walkers became "aerobically fit." At first, some couldn't walk a block, he says, but in three months they ramped up their maximum heart rates 60 to 70 percent, consistent with aerobic fitness. That meant fast-paced "aerobic walking" at a speed of about 3.5 miles an hour, or two miles in about thirty-five minutes. This may be ideal, since aerobic exercise is known to boost gray matter and neuronal fertilizers such as BDNF (brain-derived neurotropic factor) in aging brains.

Additionally, Jeffrey M. Burns, MD, a neurologist and exercise authority at the University of Kansas's Alzheimer and Memory Program, points out that older women who walked at a slow pace for only ninety minutes a week also piled up substantial cognitive benefits. It's better to walk slowly than not at all, says Burns.

What to do? Take a brisk walk every day for a total of thirty minutes or three times a week for an hour. Use a treadmill if it's easier; either go to a gym or get a treadmill for home. "Brisk" means aerobic. Here are some tips from experts on how to achieve an aerobic state. Walk as fast as you can and still carry on a conversation. Walk three to four miles in an hour. Enter a local program for "cardiovascular fitness"— synonymous with "brain fitness." Go to a gym, exercise class, personal trainer, or doctor for advice in determining the walking speed and duration you need to become aerobically fit. Remember, you can start out walking slowly and increase the pace and distance gradually. And it's okay to walk fast for ten minutes, slow down, then speed up again for another ten minutes. Three brisk ten-minute walks can be as worthwhile as a continuous thirty-minute one.

Combine walking with other brain-protecting activities for a synergistic benefit. To paraphrase Kramer: "Take a brisk walk with a good friend to talk about a book." That's a triple preventive strike against Alzheimer's. (Also see "Enjoy Exercise," page 113, "Keep Your Balance," page 40, and "Build Strong Muscles," page 198.)

100

MAKE IT **WINE**, PREFERABLY RED

Wine blocks memory loss in several ways

Wine is special—more likely than other alcoholic drinks to protect your aging brain. Once, only French and Italian researchers said it. But now Swedes and Brits and Americans and scads of other investigators endorse wine, notably red wine. Although it may still be controversial in some circles, let's just say it's odd to see a neuroscientist at a cocktail party pick up a martini, beer, or white wine over a glass of red.

Particularly compelling is a recent Swedish study of 1,462 women who were tracked for thirty-four years. The most striking finding: women who drank *only* wine and no other type of alcoholic beverages were *70 percent less* apt to develop dementia. Drinking beer and spirits conveyed no protection. Clearly, wine contains something other than alcohol that protects the brain, researchers at the University of Gothenburg concluded.

For one thing, wine, notably red wine, has antioxidants in spades. One is resveratrol, which is strongly anti-inflammatory.

Antioxidants also fight oxidative damage leading to the death of brain cells. But here's the recently discovered clincher: specific red wine antioxidants can enter living brain cells and block the deposition of Alzheimer's-inducing beta-amyloid. Such antioxidants can also improve cognition in old animals by detoxifying the existing plaques poisoning their brains, according to experiments at UCLA and Mount Sinai School of Medicine in New York.

In one test, researchers fed Alzheimer's-prone mice two types of red wine—Cabernet Sauvignon and a muscadine, both of which contain high concentrations of naturally occurring antioxidants called polyphenols. Both wines protected against and reversed brain damage—and in amounts equivalent to a mere one or two 5-ounce glasses a day! Giving the mice pure ethanol or water did not stop brain or cognitive deterioration.

Red wine has at least fifteen times more polyphenolic antioxidants than white wine, according to a recent test.

What to do? If you are already a moderate drinker, you may want to switch to red wine. *Important:* an average of one 5-ounce glass of wine a day is enough for women, two glasses for men. More can increase your risk of dementia and other diseases. If you are not a wine drinker, don't start just in hope of protecting your brain. You can get similar antioxidants by drinking lots of Concord (purple) grape juice or blueberry juice. However, it's uncertain whether they convey the same brain benefits as red wine.

PUTTING IT ALL TOGETHER:
YOUR ANTI-ALZHEIMER'S PLAN

What now? The 100 simple things to do in this book will, I trust, give you many ideas, thoughts, plans, and hopes for making your own brain stronger against forces that threaten to destroy your intellect and entire being as you grow older. And there is still much adventure ahead to keep your brain stimulated.

As bold and brilliant as they may be, our top medical minds in Alzheimer's research circles are still in mysterious territory, with ever-shifting landmarks, conflicting theories, passionate disagreements, excursions into blind alleys, and dreams of finding the precise genetic, metabolic, and pharmaceutical keys that will reveal the secrets of the disease and make interventions and cures a tested reality. It is impossible to know where exactly we are on this research journey.

My hunch is that there is still much to discover about the basic nature of beta-amyloid and tau, the role of genetics, and the thrilling potential for the regeneration of brain cells before scientists finally agree on the best ways to prevent, delay, and possibly treat age-related memory loss, dementia, and Alzheimer's.

That does not mean you should delay taking action to slash your own personal risk. Anything you do may buy you days, months, or years of memory-intact, dementia-free functioning. But nobody can yet tell you precisely what is best for you; there is no one-size-fits-all action plan, and there probably never will be.

In keeping with the spirit of how the brain thrives best, I am suggesting that you, like me, make your own action plan, incorporating ways to care for your brain and body that seem best to you. Remember, your brain cells are activated and inspired to grow only when you go off autopilot and into novelty and intellectual effort. Stirring up a billion or so lazy brain cells is what it is all about.

Here are four areas of your life where experts believe you can make the most difference in preserving cognitive functioning and pushing the symptoms of Alzheimer's beyond your life span. It's a good idea to make an action plan for each of the four areas. It appears to be never too early or too late in life to begin.

1. REV UP AND SURPRISE YOUR BRAIN

It's clear that you need to keep your awake brain on high alert, thinking and learning. The best way to get your brain's attention is by thinking and doing anything *new*. Make a list of ten new things you would like to do to engage your brain, then try them. Here's part of my list: Learn Spanish (this will be taxing; I have a record of past failures in learning any language, except Latin grammar in high school). Practice parallel parking (I am concerned about losing my depth perception). Learn to scan and organize my photographs on my computer. Go to a beginning acting class for adults. Learn to do ten to fifteen minutes of yoga meditation a day.

Make it a point to fill your leisure time with mental activities that stimulate your brain without being overly stressful. If you watch too much TV, cut back. Instead play cards or video games, attend lectures, take classes in person or on line. And try to learn something that has always been appealing but seemed too difficult. If you make a strenuous mental effort, you activate your brain, helping keep alive newborn neurons that otherwise would die from lack of stimulation. That's why learning needs to be ongoing, and the greater and longer your mental exertion, generally the better your brain likes it. Break out into new mental adventures of any type; try to think outside the box.

For inspiration, I highly recommend *The Memory Bible* and *iBrain* by Gary Small, MD, director of the UCLA Center on Aging. Using sophisticated brain scans, Small has devised techniques and mental aerobics, explained in his books, that stimulate the brain without being stressful or frustrating. Especially important, he finds that the brain becomes activated when it makes an effort to do or learn something new. When people play a computer game for the first time, PET scans show high brain activity. But as they become proficient at the game, the scans register minimal brain activity during play. Thus, you regularly need to find new mental aerobics to challenge your brain. "Look for activities or technologies that are at the right difficulty level for you," he advises. "If the game is too easy, it will not stimulate your neuronal connections and you'll get bored. If it is too challenging, you'll become frustrated and stressed."

Main message: Finding new, fun ways to exert and excite aging brain cells is key to building a resistance to Alzheimer's.

2. GET THE RIGHT TYPE AND AMOUNT OF PHYSICAL ACTIVITY

Never doubt the power of physical activity to keep your brain from being captured by the pathology and symptoms of dementia. The research is mountainous. Studies generally favor moderate aerobic exercise as the most protective. Some studies suggest that vigorous exercise is not always better than moderate exercise. And there is evidence that even a little bit of physical activity can keep you from losing your mind and memory. Being a lifetime jock may give you an edge, but it is never too late to get brain benefits from moving your body, even if only a little at first and then working up to more.

Research has yet to define a universal anti-Alzheimer's exercise plan, detailing precisely how much of what type of exercise is apt to be sufficient, and some of the research is inconsistent. In the meantime, Alzheimer's researcher Jeffery Burns, MD, at the University of Kansas says experts generally recommend at least thirty minutes of moderate aerobic exercise a day, five days a week, for a total of two and a half hours weekly. If that seems to be too much, do as much as you can. "Do fifteen minutes five days a week, and then when you get into the habit, push it up more," Burns says. Most important, he stresses, get in the habit of doing any type of physical activity daily. If it's aerobic exercise, all the better. However, he notes that many experts now declare moderate exercise of lower intensity for a longer period of time nearly as beneficial as higher-intensity, shorter-duration so-called aerobic exercise. Your brain, then, is not doomed if you fall short of the daunting pinnacle of "aerobic fitness," although the best evidence on stalling memory loss still supports that goal.

Additionally, you should include some weight training for strong muscles, exercises to maintain and improve balance, and stretching exercises for flexibility. All help reduce the risk of dementia. You can do these on your own at home, in an exercise class, or with a personal trainer. My physical activity program consists of an hour of doubles tennis three times a week, an hour at the gym twice a week, yoga once a week, and walking and dancing in between.

For a wealth of extremely helpful tips and advice on putting together an exercise plan, also take a look at the websites of the American College of Sports Medicine (www.acsm.org) and the President's Council on Physical Fitness and Sports (www.fitness.gov). The latter even gives you precise instructions for doing tests to find out your current levels of aerobic fitness, muscular strength and endurance, flexibility, and body composition. You can also directly access the tests at www.adultfitnesstest.org.

3. EAT THE RIGHT STUFF AND TAKE SUPPLEMENTS

Eating to give yourself the best odds of avoiding impaired memory or dementia means making very conscious choices. Here are fifteen suggestions of ways to eat that may help you prevent memory impairment and Alzheimer's:

- If you don't have one, get a Mediterranean-style cookbook and follow it.
- Use extra-virgin olive oil and vinegar as staples.
- Eat fatty fish, such as salmon, tuna, or sardines, twice a week or more.
- Stop eating red meat, including bacon and hot dogs, or eat it only once a month. Substitute turkey or vegetarian burgers for beef burgers.
- Drink a glass of juice every morning and as much coffee and real tea as agrees with you; if you consume alcohol, have a daily glass of wine, preferably red wine and with food. A cup or two a day of hot or cold dark chocolate—rich in flavanols and low in fat and sugar—is also good for you.
- Eat a cup of berries every day and vary them to include all types, notably blueberries, strawberries, and raspberries.
- Eat a green, orange, or other brightly colored vegetable; a green salad; and piece of fruit (such as an apple) or half a cup of fresh fruit every day.
- Eat two or three egg yolks a week.
- Eat a handful of nuts every day.

- Eat whole grains almost exclusively, including whole wheat bread, brown rice, oatmeal and other whole grain cereals, whole grain pasta, and popcorn.
- Cut way back on processed foods, especially snacks such as chips, pretzels, and crackers.
- Eat foods with a low glycemic index, to help keep blood sugar down; check a food's numbers at www.glycemicindex.com.
- Cut back on saturated and trans fats, sodium, carbohydrates, and added sugars. Read food labels carefully. Use low-fat or no-fat dairy products and/or substitute almond, soy, or rice milk.
- Restrict carbonated soft drinks (regular and diet) to a couple a month or none.
- Go for whole foods over highly processed foods. Frozen fruits and vegetables without sauces and syrups are just fine—rich in nutrients and antioxidants.

Deciding which supplements to take is a personal choice, and their effectiveness depends on many unknowns, including your current nutritional status, lifestyle, and genetic susceptibility to dementia.

Here's my take on what your priorities should be:

- At the very least, take a "once a day multivitamin" or, preferably, a multivitamin that incorporates higher doses of antioxidants.

- Be sure you are not deficient in B vitamins (notably B_{12} and folic acid) and vitamin D. If in doubt, ask your doctor for a simple blood test to detect a deficiency.
- Since so few people get enough omega-3, which is so critical for aging brains, take a fish oil supplement, whether or not you eat fatty fish.

After that, you can add whatever you want, depending on emerging evidence and your sense of your own individual needs. Here's what I generally take every day: a high-antioxidant multivitamin-mineral supplement without iron, plus whatever else is needed to make a total of 1,000 mcg B_{12}, 800 mcg folic acid, 2,000–5,000 IU vitamin D, 200 mg alpha lipoic acid, 500 mg acetyl-l-carnitine, and 400 mg DHA fish oil. It's entirely possible that new research will lead to scientifically verified cognitive-preserving and Alzheimer's-preventing formulas or drinks. Some are being developed and tested.

4. TAKE CARE OF YOURSELF

Virtually everything you do, as well as the way you feel about and act toward yourself and others, has an impact on your vulnerability to age-related memory loss and Alzheimer's symptoms. Certainly, feeling alone and isolated, without social contact and support, is a risk factor. So is being depressed, stressed, and distressed. Being easygoing and optimistic, having a wide circle of friends and family, and participating in social and community activities boost resistance to cognitive deterioration. Just as you exert yourself to be physically and mentally active, make sure you are socially active too. That may also take effort, but keep in mind that your brain loves to socialize, and human interactions encourage brain cells to flourish.

Nor does your brain live happily in isolation from the rest of your body. Its well-being is intimately connected to everything else, including your eyes, teeth, thyroid, immune system, and notably your cardiovascular system. If one part of your body falls into disrepair, your brain is apt to follow. Don't neglect routine eye and dental checkups, and pay attention to your blood pressure, blood sugar, cholesterol, and weight. Remedying such problems in middle age, as well as in later years, can dramatically reduce your likelihood of memory decline and dementia. In short, taking care of your mental and physical health helps protect your brain for a lifetime.

Is it still partly a matter of genetic luck? Absolutely, and doing everything "right" is certainly no guarantee that you will avoid the tragedy of Alzheimer's. That's why it is imperative to support the search for effective treatments as well as efforts to ameliorate the suffering of individuals and families who are living with the disease.

Still, the amazing fact is that many of us, even those close to the brink, may be able to postpone the severe symptoms of cognitive decline and dementia beyond our lifetimes by taking the advice of a growing number of Alzheimer's researchers who are rallying behind the emerging revolutionary idea that you may escape the worst of the disease by doing many of the 100 things in this book. Perhaps doing even a few of them will make a huge difference for you. As researchers predict, delaying the onset of Alzheimer's by only five years could save at least half of us from ever developing this devastating disease.

ACKNOWLEDGMENTS

I want to thank all the researchers who have sent me hundreds of their papers from leading peer-reviewed medical journals, which are the basis for this book, and for the interviews many have granted me recently as well as over the fifteen years I have been writing about aging and the brain. In particular, Gregory Cole, associate director of UCLA's Alzheimer's Disease Research Center and a leading advocate for finding ways to prevent Alzheimer's; Robert S. Wilson at Rush University Medical Center in Chicago, who has done massive amounts of research on personality and lifestyle factors that influence Alzheimer's; Patricia Boyle and Aron Buchman, also Alzheimer's researchers at Rush University, who talked with me about their research; Gary Arendash of the University of South Florida, who keeps coming up with bold, unexpected findings on possible antidotes to Alzheimer's, including caffeine; Gary Wenk at Ohio State University, who amused and informed me with his wide-ranging knowledge of research on memory and hazardous substances; Brian Balin at the Philadelphia College of Osteopathic Medicine, who brought me up-to-date on infections as a possible cause of Alzheimer's; John C. Morris, director of the Alzheimer Disease Research Center at Washington University in St. Louis and a remarkable leader in the field, with whom I share an undergraduate alma mater, Ohio Wesleyan University, and whose colleagues contribute so many new findings on preventing, detecting, diagnosing, and understanding Alzheimer's, including David Holtzman and James Galvin, who shared their latest research with me; Gary Small, director of the UCLA Center on Aging, a whirlwind of information about brain imaging and the new high-tech impact on the brain; Suzanne Tyas at the University of Waterloo in Ontario, who so generously shared her research knowledge on the famous Nun Study; Jeffrey Burns, director of the Alzheimer and Memory Program at the University of Kansas, who helped me find a consensus of expert opinion among the countless conflicting studies on physical activity and the risk of dementia; Rachel A. Whitmer of Kaiser Permanente's Division of Research in Oakland, California, who similarly helped me understand the paradox in studies on weight, body fat, and dementia; Guy Potter at Duke University Medical Center, who explained how occupation affects dementia risk; the late James Joseph, an unforgettable Tufts University researcher, who for years regaled me with his findings on the brain-protecting powers of blueberries, and with whom I served on the Board of the American Aging Association; Steven Zeisel at the University of North Carolina, who has been telling me about choline's brain-building powers for a decade; and Richard Anderson, the U.S. Department of Agriculture's pioneering researcher on diabetes, whose discoveries on the health powers of spices, such as cinnamon, have intrigued me since the 1990s.

For my basic knowledge of free radicals and antioxidants and their effects on brain aging, I am grateful to have been tutored by several remarkable pioneers in the field, with whom I have had a continuing journalistic relationship: Bruce Ames at the University of California, Berkeley; Balz Frei, director of the Linus Pauling Institute at Oregon State University; and the acknowledged "father of the free-radical theory of aging"; Denham Harman, professor emeritus at the University of Nebraska College of Medicine, who was my original mentor.

I also want to acknowledge the late Robert N. Butler, an outstanding pioneer and friend who first introduced me to the idea that Alzheimer's is not an inevitable consequence of aging when I was making a documentary on the subject for CNN. As the first director of the National Institute on Aging and founder of the International Longevity Center, Bob Butler was a monumental force in bringing the importance and promise of preventing and overcoming Alzheimer's to public prominence.

Writing this book has been on my mind for lots of years, but it would not have become a reality so quickly without the fast action of my agent, Gail Ross, in Washington, DC, who insisted on seeing a proposal as soon as she heard the idea.

Thank you, Gail. Also, there was no question of who should publish the book after I had my first conversation with Tracy Behar at Little, Brown. She understood it all instantly and has been a joy to work with. Thank you, Tracy, and everyone at Little, Brown who has so energetically and happily made the book possible.

The National Institute on Aging of the National Institutes of Health funds thirty Alzheimer's Disease Centers at major medical institutions across the country. Their mission is to find ways to cure and possibly prevent Alzheimer's and to translate the latest research into better diagnoses and care for those who develop the disease. These centers are staffed by the most prominent researchers on Alzheimer's. Their websites contain information on what's happening in the field, as well as what services they offer, such as the medical evaluation of memory problems and the diagnosis and management of Alzheimer's and other dementias. The centers also provide information on participating in drug trials, support groups, clinical research projects, and other special programs.

Alabama

University of Alabama Birmingham: 205-934-3847, www.uab.edu/adc

Arizona

Arizona Alzheimer's Disease Center/Banner Sun Health Research Institute: 602-839-6900, http://www.bannerhealth.com/Alzheimers/ Alzheimers+Institute.htm

California

University of California, Davis: 916-734-5496, http://alzheimer.ucdavis.edu

University of California, Irvine: 949-824-2382, www.alz.uci.edu

University of California, Los Angeles: Four clinics provide the most advanced diagnostic and evaluation services to patients with memory concerns. 310-794-3665, www.EastonAD.ucla.edu

University of California, San Diego: 858-622-5800, http://adrc.ucsd.edu

University of California, San Francisco: 415-476-6880, http://memory.ucsf.edu

University of Southern California: 323-442-7600, http://adrc.usc.edu

Florida
Florida Alzheimer's Disease Research Center/Byrd
Alzheimer's Institute: 866-700-7773,
www.floridaadrc.org

Georgia
Emory University: 404-728-6950,
www.med.emory.edu/ADC

Illinois
Northwestern University: 312-926-1851,
www.brain.northwestern.edu

Rush University Medical Center: 312-942-3333,
www.rush.edu/radc

Indiana
Indiana University: 317-278-5500,
http://iadc.iupui.edu

Kentucky
University of Kentucky/Alzheimer's Disease Center: 859-257-1412,
www.mc.uky.edu/coa/clinicalcore/Alzheimercenter.html

Maryland
Johns Hopkins University: 410-502-5164,
www.alzresearch.org

Massachusetts

Boston University: 888-458-2823,
www.bu.edu/alzresearch

Massachusetts General Hospital/Harvard Medical School:
617-726-3987,
http://madrc.org

Michigan

University of Michigan: 734-936-8764,
www.med.umich.edu/alzheimers

Minnesota

Mayo Clinic (jointly based in Rochester, MN, and
Jacksonville, FL): 507-284-1324,
http://mayoresearch.mayo.edu/alzheimers_center

Missouri

Washington University: 314-286-2683,
http://alzheimer.wustl.edu

New York

Columbia University: 212-305-2077,
www.alzheimercenter.org

Mount Sinai School of Medicine: 212-241-8329,
www.mssm.edu/research/centers/
alzheimers-disease-research-center

New York University: 212-263-8088,
www.med.nyu.edu/adc

North Carolina

Duke University Medical Center: 866-444-2372,
http://adrc.mc.duke.edu

Oregon

Oregon Health and Science University: 503-494-6695,
www.ohsu.edu/xd/research/centers-institutes/neurology/
alzheimers

Pennsylvania

University of Pennsylvania: 215 662 7810,
www.uphs.upenn.edu/ADC

University of Pittsburgh: 412-692-2700,
www.adrc.pitt.edu

Texas

University of Texas Southwestern Medical Center: 214-648-3239,
www.utsouthwestern.edu/alzheimers/research

Washington

University of Washington: 800-317-5382,
www.uwadrc.org

Wisconsin

University of Wisconsin: 866-636-7764,
www.wcmp.wisc.edu

A NOTE ON SCIENTIFIC REFERENCES

In writing *100 Simple Things You Can Do to Prevent Alzheimer's*, I did extensive online searches of the medical literature on PubMed, the world's largest compendium of scientific journal articles, operated by the National Institutes of Health. I also searched the websites of individual medical journals, academic research centers, government agencies, medical professional associations, major newspapers, magazines, and specialized blogs on the brain, neurology, geriatrics, and Alzheimer's. I attended online webinars and video conferences on the latest scientific investigations into the initiation, progression, diagnosis, and epidemiology of Alzheimer's and on promising interventions to delay, stop, or even reverse its pathology and symptoms.

I interviewed numerous leading Alzheimer's researchers by phone and e-mail about their findings. I also consulted many books on Alzheimer's and related topics.

The number of studies I have read and relied on for information and advice over the ten years or so I have been collecting the research on Alzheimer's prevention are in the thousands, and to list even a small fraction of them here would overwhelm the purpose and content of the book.

For readers who are interested in the major scientific references that support the information in this book, I have listed more than two hundred medical journal articles available on PubMed at my website, www.jeancarper.com. Using these references, you can look up the abstracts and articles by going to www.pubmed.gov. All abstracts, summarizing the conclusions, are free, as are some full articles. Other full articles require a fee for downloading.

INDEX

Index

excessive calories and, 60; sugar, 253
exercise lowering, 51
nicotine patch lowering, 210
as predictor of Alzheimer's or
  dementia, 33, 50–51
high blood sugar. *See* blood sugar levels
hockey, danger of brain injury in, 139
Holden, Karen, 172
Hollenberg, Norman, 64–65
Holtzman, David, 232–33
homocysteine (amino acid) levels,
  128–29, 141–42, 144–45, 196, 272
testing for, 145–46
hospitalization, effect of, 22–23
Hughes, Tiffany, 262
"hunger hormone" (leptin) deficiency,
  171–73
hypertension. *See* high blood pressure

iBrain (Small), 287
ibuprofen, 212–13
immune scavenger cells (microglia),
  153–54
India, low rate of Alzheimer's in, 83, 86
infections, brain, 95, 150–52
infection theory, 27, 150–52
inflammation, arterial, 141
inflammation, brain, 153–55
  accompanying stroke, 251
  anti-inflammatory agents, 155, 182,
    211–12; food, 167, 187, 214, 223; red
    wine, 16, 282
  B_{12} deficiency and, 272
  belly fat and, 148, 154, 277
  cholesterol and, 67
  C-reactive protein (CRP) as sign of,
    69, 142, 154, 187
  and dementia, 257–58, 265
  diabetes and, 92
  effect of, 25, 48; promotes
    Alzheimer's, 16, 148
  environmental poisons causing, 107
  exercise fighting, 148, 154
  foods fighting, 36, 44, 63, 85,
    154–55, 187

foods increasing: fast foods, 224; red
  meat, 178
gum disease and, 257
smoking and, 236
influenza virus, 151
information about Alzheimer's and
  dementia, leading sources of,
  156–58
insomnia, 58, 76, 234. *See also* sleep
  deprivation
Institute for Brain Aging and
  Dementia, 113
Institute for Memory Impairments and
  Neurological Disorders, 207
insulin dysfunction, 60, 92, 131, 159–61
  diet normalizing, 93
insulin resistance, 38, 160–61, 172;
  induced, (by belly fat) 277, (by
  sleeplessness) 233, (by sugar) 253;
  reversed, 20, (by cinnamon) 71–73,
  161, (by coffee) 75, (by cucurmin)
  86. *See also* diabetes
Internet surfing, 132–34
iron, avoidance of, 83, 197
  chelation of, 19–20, 83–84, 256;
  deposits in brain, 82–84, 179, 197
isoflurane (anesthetic), 22
Israeli studies, 169, 256
  of celiac disease, 61, 62
Italy: Alzheimer studies in, 40, 82,
  128, 222
  "smart drug" sold in, 18
Itzhaki, Ruth, 151

Japanese tea drinkers, 255
job, interesting. *See* mental stimulation
Johns Hopkins University, 47, 64, 99, 301
Joseph, James, 43, 166, 214, 239–40
Journal of Alzheimer's Disease, 150, 179
*Journal of the American Medical
  Association,* 5
juice, fruit and vegetable. *See* diet
junk food, 122–23, 224
Juvenon (lipoic acid-ALCAR pill)
  website, 20

315

Index

distress and, 102
excessive calories producing, 60
memory chemical, *see* acetylcholine
mental stimulation delaying, 193–94
nature walk restoring, 202
predictors of, 265; high homocysteine,
144
recognition of, 189–91
risk factors, 48; diabetes, 93;
environmental pollution, 107; gum
disease, 258; heart disease, 141;
oxidative damage, 179; smoking,
235–36; stress, 248–49; sugar, 253
slowed or reversed, 35–36, 44, 57, 61,
69, 85; by DASH diet, 88–89; by
nicotinamide, 206; by tea, 255–56;
by vitamin D, 274
spatial, 253
vascular dementia and, 50, 265
as warning sign, 7; short-term, 135
See also cognitive impairment
meningitis, 95
menopause, 111–12. *See also* women
"mental fluctuations," 99, 100
mental stimulation, 105–6, 132–34, 192–94
anti-Alzheimer power of, 246; and
cognitive reserve, 47–48, 77–79;
enriched environment, 245–47;
interesting job, 162–64; linguistic
skills, 168–70; novelty response,
203–5, 286–88; strength training
and, 199; video games, 266–68, 287
metabolic syndrome, 253, 278
Mevacor (statin), 243
MHCP (methylhydroxy chalcone
polymer), 72
microglia (immune scavenger cells),
153–54
micronutrients, 196
microwave, 109
ministrokes. *See* stroke
mitochondrial function, 19
Moffat, Marilyn, 41, 42
"molecular rust." *See* oxidative damage
Montine, Thomas J., 5

Morley, John E., 41, 42
Morris, John C., 8–9, 104
Morris, Martha Clare, 37, 83, 207, 239
Mortimer, James, 261
Motrin (ibuprofen), 212
Mount Sinai School of Medicine, 59, 139,
283, 302
MRI (magnetic resonance imaging),
172, 196
brain activity/inactivity shown by,
132, 134, 148, 183, 193, 271, 279–80;
sleep apnea, 220
diagnosis by, 50, 96, 265
multivitamins, 83, 195–97, 207, 291–92
muscle strength, 198–200. *See also*
exercise, physical

National Football League, 138
National Institute of Environmental
Health Sciences, 195–96
National Institutes of Health, 88, 156,
158, 185
French version (Inserm), 135;
National Institute on Aging, 25, 32,
42, 50, 60, 97, 128, 153, 157, 299;
websites, 89, 185; Women's Health
Initiative, 110–12
nature walks, 201–2. *See also* exercise,
physical
neurogenesis (brain regeneration),
46–48, 64, 114, 256
neuronal damage, 7
neuroticism (distress), 102–3
neurotoxins, 107–9, 224. *See also* beta-
amyloid (brain toxin);
environmental toxins; iron deposits
in brain; tau (brain toxin)
Newberg, Andrew, 184
Newhouse, Paul A., 209–10
New Mexico studies, 197
New York University, 41, 303
Langone Medical Center, 189
niacin (vitamin B_3), 136–37, 206–8
nicotinamide, 197, 206–8
nicotine patch, 209–10, 236

nitric oxide, 89
nitrosamines, dangers of, 179
Northwestern University, Cognitive
Neurology and Alzheimer's Disease
Center, 22, 301
Norwegian cola study, 136
No Sweat Exercise Plan, The (Simon), 116
novelty response, 203–5, 286–88. *See also*
mental stimulation
NSAIDs (non-steroidal anti-
inflammatory drugs), 211–13. *See
also* drugs, nonprescription
Nun Study, 47, 168–69, 242
nuts, 30, 79, 89, 136, 290; peanuts, 131,
207; walnuts and almonds, 214–16

obesity, 6, 60, 92
as Alzheimer's risk factor/predictor, 33,
196; and brain shrinkage, 48, 217–18;
defined by body mass index (BMI),
217, 262, 276; diet preventing, 86,
130; and leptin resistance, 172, 173;
middle-age, concern about, 217–19;
sleeplessness and, 233; and sudden
weight loss, 262; sugar and, 253;
visceral, *see* belly fat
"obesity paradox," 218–19, 277
oleocanthal (organic compound), 222–23
oligomers, 223, 227. *See also* beta-
amyloid (brain toxin)
oil, olive, 38, 187–88, 222–23, 225, 290;
other acceptable oils, 223
omega-3 oil, 34, 38, 48, 125, 154, 173, 187
diet sources of, 126; diet supplements,
292
protection reduced by omega-6, 225
omega-6 fat, 126, 154, 224–25
orange juice, 167, 274–75
Oregon Health and Science University,
47, 303
oxidative damage, 19, 29, 60, 107, 179,
214. *See also* antioxidants

PAD (peripheral artery disease), 24,
141, 143

Pagnoni, Giuseppe, 183
Parkinson's disease, 7, 179
pedometer, use of, 149. *See also* exercise,
physical
periodontal problems. *See* teeth
peripheral artery disease. *See* PAD
personality traits, 101–3
pesticides, 107–9
PET (positron-emission tomography)
scans, 8, 77–78, 96, 104, 193, 226, 287
Petersen, Ronald, 134
pharmaceuticals. *See* drugs, prescription
Philadelphia College of Osteopathic
Medicine, 27, 150
physical activity. *See* exercise, physical
physical inactivity (sedentary lifestyle),
6, 92, 142, 147–49, 196
and resistance exercise, 199
plaques and tangles, 226–28, 238, 250.
See also beta-amyloid (brain toxin);
tau (brain toxin)
plastic containers, 109
pneumonia, community-acquired, 150
pollution, 107–9, 196
polyphenols, 166, 283. *See also*
antioxidants
pomegranate juice, 165–67
Posit Science website, 133
potassium, value of, 251
Potter, Guy, 162
poultry, 39, 180, 188, 207
pregnancy: and diet, 58, 68, 69; caffeine,
76. *See also* women
President's Council on Physical Fitness
and Sports website, 115
preventive intervention, 5, 8–10, 33,
142, 191
diet and, 29, 43, 60, 86, 89, 130,
165–67; olive oil, 223
education and, 105; linguistic skills,
168–70 (*see also* mental stimulation)
exercise, 148 (*see also* exercise,
physical)
NSAIDs, 212–13
prostaglandins, 224

Jean Carper is an award-winning medical journalist who specializes in nutrition. She is the author of twenty-three books, including the *New York Times* bestsellers *Food: Your Miracle Medicine, Stop Aging Now!* and *Miracle Cures,* along with *Your Miracle Brain* and *Jean Carper's Complete Healthy Cookbook.* She is a contributing editor to *USA Weekend* magazine and wrote the magazine's "EatSmart" column for fourteen years.

Carper was the first senior medical correspondent for CNN, where she won a prestigious ACE Award for her series on brain cancer. She has also received excellence in journalism awards from the American Aging Association and the American College of Nutrition, and she has served on the boards of the American Aging Association and the American Botanical Council.

A graduate of Ohio Wesleyan University, she is a recipient of the university's lifetime achievement award. She lives in Washington, DC, and Florida.